HandGuyMD® Patient Guide:

Carpal Tunnel Syndrome

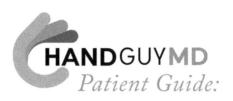

HANDGUY**MD**
Patient Guide:

CARPAL TUNNEL
SYNDROME

HELP FOR YOUR HANDS

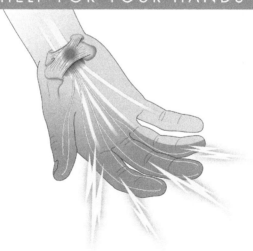

WREN V. McCALLISTER, MD, MBA

MILL CITY PRESS

Mill City Press, Inc.
2301 Lucien Way #415
Maitland, FL 32751
407.339.4217
www.millcitypress.net

Illustrations (cover and interior) by Lisa May

The information included in this book is for educational purposes only. It is not intended or implied to be a substitute for professional medical advice. The reader should always consult his or her healthcare provider to determine the appropriateness of the information for his or her own situation or if he or she has any questions regarding a medical condition or treatment plan. Reading the information in this book does not constitute a physician patient relationship. The author and publisher expressly disclaim responsibility for any adverse effects that may result from the use or application of the information contained in this book.

Edited by Mill City Press.

Paperback ISBN-13: 9781662842627
eBook ISBN-13: 9781662842634

To the many thousands of patients that I have been privileged to meet over the years: I am deeply appreciative of the trust you have placed in me and my team.

We are honored to be a part of your musculoskeletal healthcare journey, helping you regain function and get back to doing what is important to you.

CONTENTS

PREFACE

As a busy practicing hand surgeon, I regularly encounter patients suffering from the signs and symptoms of carpal tunnel syndrome (CTS). While not every patient with CTS needs surgery, those who do often tell me that they had been suffering the symptoms for a long time before seeking any treatment. This may explain why the condition progressed to the point where nonoperative treatment was no longer successful. The right information at the right time may have prevented the condition from progressing. A core philosophy I hold is that empowering patients with trusted information results in better healthcare. You are to be congratulated for taking action to improve your health.

This book is a guide to help you understand what it means when you are diagnosed with carpal tunnel syndrome; the signs and symptoms associated with carpal tunnel syndrome; how to interact with your providers; and a description of steps you can take to reduce or eliminate symptoms you may be experiencing. The information in this book will help you at any stage: to avoid developing symptoms; reversing symptoms if you are experiencing numbness and tingling; or preventing their recurrence—but only if you act.

This book is not a consultation with a hand surgeon. Every individual is different with specific signs, symptoms and a unique medical history. I cannot know the specific details of your situation without meeting you in person. I do regularly encounter patients who present with symptoms, thinking they have carpal tunnel syndrome (and they do not), and others who have ignored the numbness and tingling for years before seeking medical attention. In both cases, accurate information about what carpal tunnel syndrome is, and what it isn't, would improve the quality of their lives. It is my hope that the information and education provided in this book will serve as a guide to help increase your understanding and start you on the path toward improved health.

The clinic visit today is an imperfect experience for patients. There is a lot of information that gets communicated in a short amount of time. Studies show that patients only retain a small portion of what was communicated during a typical visit. This book will help to fill in the blanks and allow you to develop a greater understanding of CTS. This means better compliance with treatment and an improved outcome.

Specifically, the HandGuyMD® Patient Guide: Carpal Tunnel Syndrome will help you:

↻ Increase your understanding of the condition, its treatment, and prevention.

↻ Improve the quality of your interaction with treating providers.

↻ Understand an evidence-based *treatment program* used with thousands of patients over two decades.

↻ Understand an evidence-based *prevention program* to minimize the risk of developing the symptoms of CTS or their recurrence.

How should you use this book? This book is designed as a guide, providing information and progressing in a logical manner. Because we are dealing with a subject that is often described in an unusual language (the language of medicine), I have tried to quickly define terms in easy-to-understand language as they appear in the text. A glossary is also included at the end. The liberal use of figures and diagrams also helps to communicate important concepts and further improve understanding.

Section I explains what CTS is and what it isn't and discusses the history of the condition, what it means to have CTS, how you may have acquired CTS, and what the evidence suggests is happening anatomically when you have CTS. Section II discusses how we determine if a patient has CTS, as well as what symptoms, physical exam findings, and tests are helpful in making that determination. The understanding you gain will significantly improve any interaction you have with a healthcare provider by reducing the confusion and stress commonly associated with an office visit. Section III focuses on how we treat CTS with a complete discussion of the range of available treatment options. Starting with nonoperative treatment and progressing all the way to surgery, this information will help you understand what is being recommended and why. There is a focus on evidence-based medicine and discussion of the AAOS/ASSH Clinical Practice Guideline for the Treatment of Carpal Tunnel Syndrome (the guidelines are explained in the chapter). In addition, there is a complete discussion of the surgery and the recovery after surgery that will reduce confusion and anxiety surrounding this treatment option that is frequently needed to resolve the condition. Finally, Section IV is aimed at preventing symptoms from either occurring or recurring, relying on the best evidence to guide us about what steps to take.

There is a tremendous volume of information available about CTS and, with the growth of the Internet, much of it is unfiltered, leaving patients without the ability to put it into perspective. **HandGuyMD®** serves as a filter and consolidator to help you make sense of the overwhelming amount of information you can access about CTS. Just as I treasure the opportunity to have a positive impact on my patients' lives every day in my hand surgery practice, my hope in writing this book is to provide you with the information and education you need to improve the quality of your life. Please feel free to reach out and let me know how this book has helped you; I welcome any suggestions for ways to increase the value you receive in the next edition. You can visit our website (www.HandGuyMD.com) or send an e-mail to DrWren@ HandGuyMD.com.

I wish you the best in achieving better health through empowered action using trusted information.

Wren V. McCallister, MD, MBA
Edmonds, Washington
August 2021

HANDGUYMD®

What is **HandGuyMD®**? In the medical community, we often refer to each other by the specialty in which we focus our practices. In orthopedics, I am often referred to as the "Hand Guy" because of my focus on surgery of the hand and upper extremity. Referring providers in my community will say to their patients, "I want you to go see the Hand Guy, Dr. McCallister." When I meet administrators or other doctors, we will introduce ourselves by our specialties, "Hi, my name is Dr. McCallister, and I am the Hand Guy." Well, **HandGuyMD®** is where you can now go to get *"Expert Help for Hand Problems."*

HandGuyMD® is an online resource focused specifically on conditions affecting the hand and upper extremity. **HandGuyMD®** enables people to improve the quality of their lives by providing trusted information and education in the personalized manner that best matches their own unique learning preferences. You get the time you need to understand the information and can revisit it as often as you need to—no longer will you remain confused after visiting with your doctor or not get all the information you needed because you forgot to ask something. **HandGuyMD®** provides a path to optimal outcomes by improving your understanding of diagnosis, treatment and prevention.

With the ever-expanding amount of information on the Internet, **HandGuyMD®** acts as a filter and serves as a resource to help you. There are many generic websites that promise to provide symptom checkers and information about various medical conditions. They are trying to be all things to all people and often only provide the most generic information about specific conditions—the clutter that is the Internet unfiltered. **HandGuyMD®** is different: it is a laser-focused resource that has the perspective of a specialist. **HandGuyMD®** will guide you with the same expert information and education that patients receive in an office visit with a hand surgeon specialist.

SECTION I

WHAT IS CARPAL TUNNEL SYNDROME?

CARPAL TUNNEL SYNDROME

Signs—Objective evidence of a disease condition identified by direct physical examination of the patient.

Symptoms—Subjective evidence suggesting the presence of a disease condition that is reported by the patient.

Median nerve—One of three major nerves that supply the hand. It provides sensation for the thumb, index, middle, and one-half of the ring finger (see figure 2).

Carpal tunnel syndrome (CTS) is the name given to the collection of signs and symptoms that result when the median nerve is under too much pressure within the carpal tunnel. The carpal tunnel is the part of the wrist that acts as the passageway for tendons and the median nerve to enter the hand (see figure 1). Carpal tunnel syndrome (CTS) is the most common cause of compressive neuropathy in the upper extremity and affects an estimated 8 million Americans each year and many millions more worldwide.[1] In the United States alone, the cost of medical care related to CTS is estimated to be $2 billion annually.[2] The prevalence of carpal tunnel

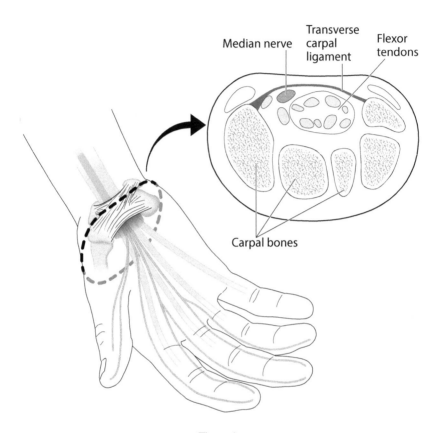

Figure 1
The Carpal Tunnel
The median nerve lies within the carpal tunnel at the level of the wrist. The carpal bones form the "floor" of the tunnel, and the "roof" is the transverse carpal ligament. The flexor tendons also occupy space within the carpal tunnel.

syndrome is estimated at 1% of the general population and 5% of the at-risk working population.[3] According to the American Academy of Orthopedic Surgeons 2016 Clinical Practice Guideline Update, between 1997 and 2010, CTS was the second most common cause of workplace absenteeism with individuals missing between 21 and 32 days of work.[4]

When the nerve becomes compressed or pinched within the carpal tunnel, the initial result is tingling, and sometimes pain, in the hand and fingers (see figure 2). These symptoms tend to occur in a predictable pattern along the distribution of the median nerve. Patients may describe an electrical-like shock that spreads to the hand and fingers.

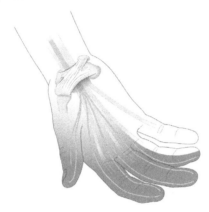

Figure 2
Median Nerve Sensory Distribution
The median nerve is responsible for sensation to the thumb, index, middle, and ½ of the ring finger (shaded area).

As the condition progresses, pain can spread up into the forearm and weakness can develop, as the muscles of the hand atrophy (see figure 3). The combination of muscle atrophy and numbness can make even the simplest tasks, like buttoning a shirt, challenging.

Atrophy—Muscle wasting that results from lack of use. This can occur either when the nerve that supplies the muscle is damaged, and thus cannot send messages to the muscle (as in CTS), or when the muscle is immobilized to prevent its use (for example, to protect a healing injury).

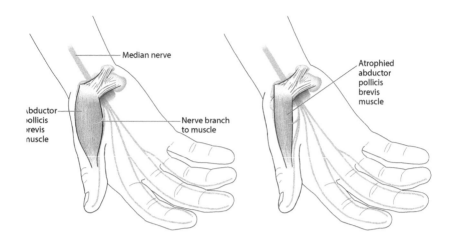

Figure 3
Thenar Muscle Atrophy
A branch of the median nerve (recurrent motor branch) exits the end of the carpal tunnel
and supplies the abductor pollicis brevis muscle. When CTS progress, this nerve branch
is affected and loses its ability to supply the muscle—leading to wasting and atrophy.

In many patients we diagnose with carpal tunnel syndrome, we cannot identify a specific cause for their symptoms (so-called idiopathic carpal tunnel syndrome). Despite a tremendous amount of research, there is no established cause-and-effect

Idiopathic—How we describe a disease condition that arises spontaneously, or for which the cause is unknown.

relationship that directly defines carpal tunnel syndrome. There are many conditions associated with carpal tunnel syndrome, and many occupations that appear to have a higher prevalence of carpal tunnel syndrome when compared to the population. Based on the recent American Academy of Orthopedic Surgeons 2016 Clinical Practice Guideline Update, it appears that there is a strong association between body-mass index (BMI), wrist anatomy, and repetitive forceful gripping and CTS.[4]

There is no one true gold standard for diagnosing CTS. Because CTS is so prevalent in the population, and our activities are so varied, it is difficult to produce good evidence that definitively identifies causes, risk factors, and specific diagnostic tools for CTS.

RISK FACTORS FOR DEVELOPING CTS

The best evidence suggests that the risk of developing carpal tunnel syndrome has the strongest association with (1) a high body-mass index (BMI) and (2) a high hand or wrist repetition rate, which is often associated with forceful, repetitive gripping with the wrist in non-neutral positions (in other words, the wrist is flexed or extended while exerting the force).[4,5,6]

Table 1 lists some of the many other conditions that have evidence suggesting an association with the increased risk of developing carpal tunnel syndrome.[4]

TABLE 1
Probable Risk Factors for Developing CTS

℃ Tendonitis (affecting wrist and/or hand)

℃ Wrist ratio/index (basically a measure of how small your wrist is at the carpal tunnel)

℃ Psychosocial factors

℃ Pregnancy

℃ Peri-menopause

℃ Inflammatory arthritis (for example, rheumatoid arthritis)

℃ Gardening

℃ Assembly line work

℃ Medical conditions (for example, acromegaly and mucopolysaccharidosis)

℃ Computer work

℃ Exposure of the hand and wrist to vibration

℃ Forceful repetitive gripping/exertion in the workplace

Table 2 lists some of the conditions that have less strong evidence for being risk factors associated with the development of CTS.[4] This means that the evidence isn't as strong, but there may be an association that has not yet been proven.

TABLE 2
Possible Risk Factors for Developing CTS

Ĉ Kidney dialysis

Ĉ Fibromyalgia

Ĉ Varicosis (veins swelling in the limb)

Ĉ Distal radius fracture (broken wrist)

Table 3 lists risk factors that have conflicting evidence for an association with developing CTS.[4]

TABLE 3
May or May Not be Risk Factors for Developing CTS

Ĉ Diabetes

Ĉ Gender

Ĉ Genetic profile (family history)

Ĉ Drug use associated with other medical conditions

Ĉ Smoking

Ĉ Bending the wrist without force or repetition

Moderate evidence shows that the use of oral contraception and female hormone replacement therapy are not risk factors for developing CTS.[4] It also appears that race or ethnicity are not independent risk factors nor is the level of a female's education.[4]

Finally, there is moderate evidence that physical activity and exercise are associated with a *decreased* risk of developing CTS.[4]

Please be aware that the presence of CTS does not mean that you have any of the conditions listed in the tables. We sometimes observe a greater incidence of CTS in patients who have these conditions when compared to patients without these conditions. The challenge comes when applying scientific principles to tease out causal relationships. Because CTS is such a common condition and has many potential factors affecting its development, it is difficult to design research studies that can establish causation.

> **Incidence**—The frequency with which a disease occurs in a population.

Regardless of whether we can establish an association, the result of any potential cause is compression of, and pressure on or within, the median nerve. This can occur if something is putting pressure on the nerve from outside the nerve (a mass or swelling in the carpal tunnel, tendon lining swelling, bony overgrowths, unusual muscles, etc.), if there is a problem with the nerve itself that leads to swelling from within the nerve (a nerve tumor or inflammation of the nerve), or if there are certain activities that repeatedly result in pressure on the nerve and produce thickening or scarring of the nerve.

Chapter 1 Summary

🍂 Carpal tunnel syndrome (CTS) is the name given to the collection of signs and symptoms that result when the median nerve is under too much pressure within the carpal tunnel.

🍂 CTS is the most common cause of compressive neuropathy in the upper extremity, affecting an estimated 8 million Americans each year and many millions more worldwide.

🍂 In the United State alone, the cost of medical care related to CTS is estimated to be $2 billion annually.

🍂 The prevalence of CTS is estimated at 1% of the general population and 5% of the at-risk working population.

🍂 Between 1997 and 2010, CTS was the second most common cause of workplace absenteeism, with individuals missing between 21 and 32 days.

🍂 When the nerve is under pressure within the carpal tunnel, the initial result is tingling and sometimes pain and weakness in the hand and fingers along the distribution of the median nerve.

🍂 Despite a tremendous amount of research, there is no established cause- and-effect relationship that directly defines carpal tunnel syndrome. However, there are many conditions associated with carpal tunnel syndrome and many occupations that appear to have a higher prevalence of carpal tunnel syndrome, when compared to the population.

ℭ Risk factors for developing CTS: The best evidence suggests that the risk of developing carpal tunnel syndrome has the strongest association with (1) a high body-mass index (BMI) and (2) a high hand or wrist rate of repetitive movement, which is often associated with forceful, repetitive gripping with the wrist in non-neutral positions.

SUPPLEMENT

WHAT DO NERVES DO?

When the median nerve is affected by CTS, whether by pressure from outside the nerve, within the nerve, or due to nerve scarring, it loses its ability to efficiently conduct nerve impulses. Nerves are designed to carry signals between our command center (our brain) and the various parts of our bodies (like fingers or toes) and organs (like the heart, lungs, kidneys, etc.). The nerves function as two-way streets and send signals from our parts (fingers, toes, organs) back to our command center (brain) for processing (see figure 4). This is a complex process, but you can think of nerves as a communication network that allows us to interact with our environment and monitor our internal functioning. When there are problems with the nerves, predictable consequences can result. For example, if you cut a nerve to your finger, you will not be able to feel the part of your finger supplied by that nerve (see figure 5).

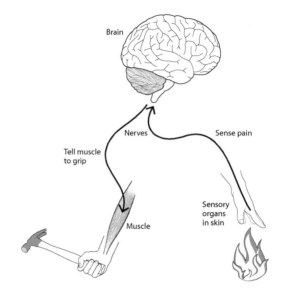

Figure 4
What Do Nerves Do?
Our brain is the command center and nerves are the "highway system" our bodies use to transport information both to and from our brains. Without nerves, we cannot process information from our environment, nor can we initiate interaction with our environment.

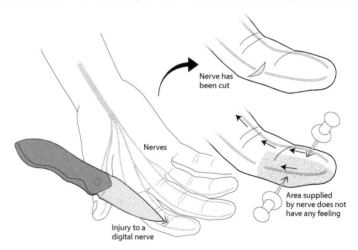

Figure 5
What Happens When You Cut a Nerve?
When you cut a nerve, you disrupt the transport of signals from that nerve at the level of the injury. That means your command center (brain) cannot receive information or send signals to anything on the other side of the injury—the road and all traffic using it is blocked.

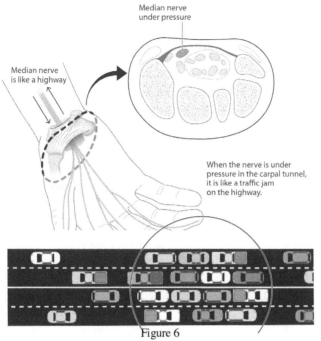

Median nerve under pressure

Median nerve is like a highway

When the nerve is under pressure in the carpal tunnel, it is like a traffic jam on the highway.

Figure 6
The Carpal Tunnel "Traffic Jam"
You can think of the median nerve as functioning like a highway and when traffic is freely flowing, there are no problems. But when the traffic slows down, the nerve begins to show signs of what we call CTS. When we use electrodiagnostic testing to measure the nerve's ability to conduct an impulse, we can quantify the degree of slowing. The goal of treatment for CTS is to free up this traffic jam and get the nerve once again flowing freely.

If your nerve is pinched somewhere along the way, you can think of it much like when there is an accident on the freeway and traffic is backed up (see figure 6). This nerve "traffic jam" has consequences: you may not be able to feel sensations as easily, or it may require more pressure to grip something before you can tell you are holding it. When the nerve "traffic jam" starts to form, often the earliest sign is tingling in the part of the body that is supplied by that nerve. As the "traffic jam" worsens, the ability of that nerve to function becomes increasingly impaired. At some point, the nerve may stop working—even if you can clear the "traffic jam" (that is, relieve the pressure).

Because the nerve is part of a complex communication network, when a person experiences signs or symptoms of nerve dysfunction, it is important to identify where along this network the problem is located. More than one problem with a nerve can give you the same symptoms, making it critical to accurately solve this puzzle and localize the source of nerve dysfunction (see figure 7). Sometimes this is easy to do, and in other cases it can be harder to distinguish or there may indeed be two separate causes for the same symptom.

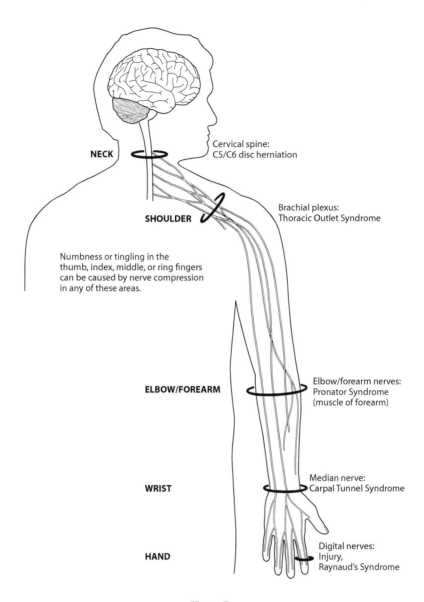

NECK

Cervical spine:
C5/C6 disc herniation

SHOULDER

Brachial plexus:
Thoracic Outlet Syndrome

Numbness or tingling in the
thumb, index, middle, or ring fingers
can be caused by nerve compression
in any of these areas.

ELBOW/FOREARM

Elbow/forearm nerves:
Pronator Syndrome
(muscle of forearm)

WRIST

Median nerve:
Carpal Tunnel Syndrome

HAND

Digital nerves:
Injury,
Raynaud's Syndrome

Figure 7
Where the Median Nerve is at Risk
Symptoms (numbness and tingling) are the result of nerve dysfunction. There are many
places along the course of a nerve where it can have trouble. For the median nerve,
symptoms in the hand could be caused by trouble at the neck, shoulder area, forearm,
wrist, or in the fingers. Diagnosis is the process of determining where the trouble
is located.

2

BRIEF HISTORY OF
CARPAL TUNNEL SYNDROME

One of the earliest descriptions of what we now know as CTS was written by Sir James Paget in 1854.[7] In his *Lectures on Surgical Pathology*, Paget described the clinical findings and pathologic anatomy of two patients in whom he believed the median nerve was injured. The first was a male who had a cord wrapped around his wrist, leading to pain, decreased sensation, and ulcerations on the back of his hand. Seven years later, his arm was amputated, and as he dissected the amputated limb, he noted:

> "...the median nerve, where it passes under the annular ligament, is enlarged with adhesions to all the adjacent tissues, and induration of both it and them [sic]".[7]

> **Tardy median nerve palsy**—The term used when the onset of median nerve dysfunction is delayed or occurs some time later after an injury.

A second patient, also a male, developed a tardy median nerve palsy after a fracture of the distal radius. About this patient, Paget wrote:

"He had ulcerations of the thumb, fore, and middle fingers, which resisted various treatment and was cured only by so binding the wrist that the parts on the palmar aspect being relaxed, the pressure on the nerve became and remained well, but as soon as the man was allowed to use his hand, the pressure on the nerve was renewed, and the ulcerations of the parts supplied by them returned."

The accounting of this second patient amounts to one of the first descriptions of wrist splinting in the neutral position, which remains today one of the most important steps in the treatment of CTS.

In 1880 the neurologist James Putnam published what is likely the first description of the major symptoms of CTS: nighttime numbness, tingling, and pain.[8] He described 37 patients with pain and paresthesias in the distribution of the median nerve, all of whom had nocturnal (nighttime) or early-morning numbness that led to pain and was relieved by hanging, shaking, or otherwise rubbing the hands. Interestingly, he also advocated several treatments for the condition that included galvanism, strychnine, and cannabis indica. However, beyond suggesting these treatments,

> **Paresthesias**—An abnormal sensation, often described as a prickling or tingling feeling (pins and needles), because of pressure on, or damage to, a peripheral nerve.

he did not report if they were successful in reducing symptoms.

The symptoms described by Putnam became known at the time as "Putnam's paresthesia,"[8] and in 1893, German neurologist Friedrich Schultze both confirmed the sensory findings reported by Putnam and coined a new term for them: acroparesthesia.[9] Then in 1908, Hunt published the first report of thenar muscle atrophy due to compression of the motor branch of the median nerve.[10] In so doing, he did not report or consider the sensory symptoms in his patients and, as a result, for many years the focus was only on motor changes. Patients who presented with both sensory and

> **Brachial Plexus**—A network of nerves formed from parts of the lower cervical (neck) nerves and the first thoracic (chest) nerve. The collection of nerves rearranges within the brachial plexus, and they emerge to enter the arm as the major named nerves in the extremity (radial, median, ulnar, musculocutaneous).

motor findings were diagnosed with a compression of the brachial plexus due to a cervical rib. This was significant because from about 1910 to 1940, the main treatment for patients with both sensory and motor findings of median nerve compression was cervical rib excision. After a couple, of decades, people began to figure out that this treatment didn't work well and re-examined the basic pathophysiology of CTS.

The continued effort to understand what was happening in patients with symptoms of CTS resulted in a 1913 publication by Marie and Foix, who wrote the first comprehensive histopathological and anatomical study of an atraumatic median nerve lesion.[11] They described findings at autopsy of an 80-year-old female whose median nerve had an "hourglass configuration with nodular thickening, then constriction at the annular ligament." This was an elegant description of the median nerve being compressed within the carpal tunnel. The hourglass shape results when the nerve becomes pinched within the carpal tunnel. There is then a resulting swelling of the nerve at the entry and exit to the carpal tunnel (see figure 8).

They also suggested a treatment for this condition: "If diagnosed early, transection of the ligament could stop the development of these phenomena." This would turn out to be an early and accurate description of the definitive treatment of CTS; however, it was largely ignored for the next twenty years, thus slowing progress in the treatment of CTS.

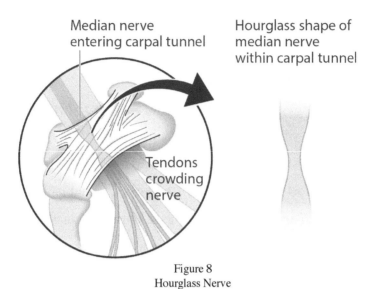

Median nerve entering carpal tunnel

Hourglass shape of median nerve within carpal tunnel

Tendons crowding nerve

Figure 8
Hourglass Nerve
When the median nerve is under mechanical pressure within the carpal tunnel, it can deform and change shape. It takes on an "hourglass" shape because of the relative tightness within the carpal tunnel. This hourglass shape corresponds to slowing of nerve function and clinical symptoms in the hand.

In the 1920s and thereafter, the investigative momentum began to pick up, and many authors were describing the condition of CTS. In 1922, Lewis and Miller wrote about CTS after a fracture of the distal radius.[12] Watson-Jones, in 1929, described CTS associated with a dislocation of the carpus[5], while Abbott and Saunders in 1933 reported chronic CTS after a fracture in the distal forearm.[13] These publications and others began to focus attention on the many possible traumatic causes of median nerve compression.

As first suggested by Marie and Foix in 1913, the surgical treatment of CTS was relatively straightforward: release the ligament and, thereby, the compression on the median nerve in the carpal tunnel. While Herbert Galloway is credited with performing the first formal open carpal tunnel release in 1924[14], it was Learmonth in 1933 who published the first detailed description of what remains today the definitive treatment for CTS: release of the transverse carpal ligament.[15] He wrote:

> *"The median nerve was exposed at the wrist joint. It was compressed between the anterior annular ligament and the arthritic outgrowths of the carpal bones. Scissors were passed under the skin so that one blade was superficial and the other deep to the annular ligament, which was then divided completely."*

Today, there are many ways to perform this operation, but they all share the same fundamental concept first described by Learmonth: dividing the transverse carpal ligament at the carpal tunnel (see figure 9).

Up until the late 1930s, much of the published literature describing compression of the median nerve focused on its occurrence after trauma or injury. Around this time, people began reporting cases of median nerve compression that occurred without any associated trauma. In 1938 Moersch wrote about a syndrome later in life involving thenar atrophy and, *"in some instances paresthesias and even sensory changes"*.[16] In 1947, Brain, Wright, and Wilkinson published a description of six patients with "spontaneous" CTS who had, *"initial burning and tingling…in the distribution of the median nerve…thenar muscle weakness…waste fairly rapidly."*[17]

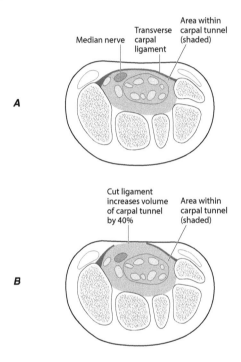

Figure 9
Dividing the Transverse Carpal Ligament
Surgical treatment of CTS requires complete division of the transverse carpal ligament (A). When this is done, the relative volume within the carpal tunnel increases by about 40% and the pressure on the nerve is relieved (B).

It was Phalen, in 1950, who finally brought it all together with his description of CTS as a clinical syndrome that resulted from compression of the median nerve at the wrist.[18] Phalen emphasized the diagnosis of CTS using sensory and motor findings and recommended splinting and injections as nonoperative treatments. He reported on three patients treated surgically (all of whom experienced immediate relief) and described use of the "Tinel's sign" for diagnosis of carpal tunnel syndrome (see figure 10).

> **Tinel's sign**—A way to identify nerves that are irritated. The examiner taps over the nerve and, if it is positive, the patient will feel a tingling sensation along the distribution of the nerve.

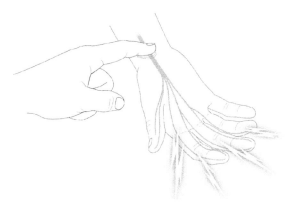

Figure 10
Tinel's Sign
A Tinel's sign results when the examiner taps the area over an irritated nerve and the patient experiences an electrical-like shock sensation along the course of the nerve.

Later, in 1966, Phalen would describe another physical exam sign when he commented that *"the numbness and paresthesias in the fingers of these patients could be increased by flexing the wrist for a period of 60 seconds. Prompt improvement in these symptoms would result with release of the wrist from the flexed position."*[19] This would become known as "Phalen's sign" (see figure 11).

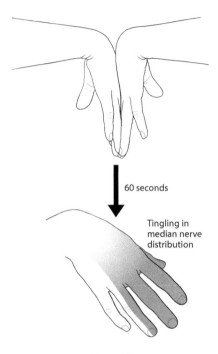

60 seconds

Tingling in
median nerve
distribution

Figure 11
Phalen's Sign

Phalen's sign is said to be positive when a patient experiences numbness and tingling in the distribution of the median nerve after 30 to 60 seconds of maintaining the wrist in a flexed position. This test has a relatively high false-positive rate (meaning that a patient will experience symptoms and a "positive test" when they do not have CTS).

By 1960, CTS was a well-defined entity with a clear treatment pathway. As a result, it became an easily diagnosed and treated condition. Today, it remains the most commonly diagnosed peripheral nerve entrapment neuropathy.

Peripheral nerve entrapment neuropathy— Just a fancy way to say that a nerve is pinched somewhere after it leaves the spinal cord. Usually this pinching occurs somewhere along the nerve's path as it travels within the arm or leg.

Chapter 2 Summary

    First described in the mid-1800s, CTS was recognized as contributing to hand dysfunction and the early descriptions of nighttime numbness, tingling, and pain are consistent with our present-day understanding of CTS.

    A 1913 publication by Marie and Foix was the first comprehensive histopathological and anatomical study of an atraumatic median nerve lesion. They also suggested a treatment for this condition: *"If diagnosed early, transection of the ligament could stop the development of these phenomena."*[11]

    While Herbert Galloway is credited with performing the first formal open carpal tunnel release in 1924, it was Learmonth in 1933 who published the first detailed description of what remains today the definitive treatment for CTS: release of the transverse carpal ligament.[14, 15]

    Phalen, in 1950, finally tied everything together with his description of CTS as a clinical syndrome that resulted from compression of the median nerve at the wrist.

    By 1960, CTS was a well-defined entity with a clear treatment pathway. As a result, it became an easily diagnosed and treated condition. Today, it remains the most commonly diagnosed peripheral entrapment neuropathy.

HOW COMMON IS CARPAL TUNNEL SYNDROME & WHO GETS IT?

t is estimated that the incidence of CTS is 99 to 148 per 100,000 people.[20] This means that out of every 100,000 people, between 99 and 148 will have CTS. The prevalence of CTS ranges from 3% to 5% in the general population and is slightly higher within the working population (8%).[2, 21] That means that at any point in time between 3% and 8% of the population may have symptoms of CTS.

In certain occupations, the prevalence is even higher, ranging from 17% to 61%.[22] These occupations tend to involve forceful repetitive hand motions in non-neutral wrist positions. Examples of such occupations include butchers, grinders, grocery-store workers, frozen-food factory workers, etc. (see figure 12).

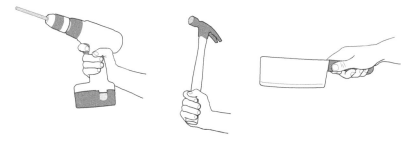

Construction worker / Carpenter   **Butcher / Meat Cutter**

Figure 12
Occupations at Risk for CTS
Workers in occupations that involve repetitive wrist motion with forceful gripping are at
the highest risk for developing CTS. Some examples include construction workers, meat
cutters and grocery store workers

CTS appears to become more common as we age, with an estimated 82% of cases occurring in patients over 40 years old. Females represent 65% to 75% of cases, and in 60% to 70% of cases CTS occurs in both hands.[23]

It is estimated that between 400,000 to 600,000 surgeries for CTS are performed each year in the United States. In 2006, there were 577,000 surgeries performed to treat CTS, which represented a 38% increase over the number of surgeries from the prior decade.[24] The total economic cost of treating CTS in 1995 was estimated at $2 billion and these costs undoubtedly higher today. Furthermore, the cost of care is affected by whether the condition developed at work. The cost of care for patients with active workmen's compensation claims costs is *three times* the cost of care provided to workers without an active workmen's compensation claim and *five times* the cost of treating non-workers.[20] The average time-off from work for patients is 28 days, and the resulting economic cost can exceed $90,000 per individual.[25]

Because CTS is an accepted occupational disease and arises more frequently in persons working in certain occupations, there is a lot of confusion about the symptoms of CTS and their relationship to work. To identify risk factors, a review of 22 epidemiologic studies was completed. The various risk factors identified had odds-ratios ranging from 1.7 to 34. The strongest conclusions from the review are shown in Table 4.[26]

Odds-ratio—A measure of the association between an exposure (think of risk factor) and an outcome. The odds-ratio tells you the odds (or chances) that an outcome will occur, given a specific exposure compared to the odds (or chances) that the same outcome would occur without the specific exposure. For example, an odds-ratio of 3 for keyboarding means that you are three times more likely to develop CTS if you keyboard than you would if you did not keyboard.

TABLE 4
Risk Factors for CTS Based on Scientific Evidence

- Repetitive motion with the hand and wrist
- Forceful motion with the hand and wrist
- Non-neutral wrist position while performing activities
- Cold temperatures (though the studies did not control for force and repetitive motion)
- Synergistic relationship between two or more risk factors

Synergistic relationship—
The idea that while the risk of developing CTS in the presence of any one individual risk factor may be small, when you start to add two or more risk factors, the relative risk of developing CTS is greater than the sum of the individual risks. In other words, $1 + 1 > 2$.

Dose response effect—
The idea that the greater your exposure to the risk factor, the greater the risk of developing CTS: little exposure, little risk and high exposure, high risk. This is a fundamental criterion for establishing causality in medicine.

It has been suggested that a dose response effect is also involved, but this has yet to be proved conclusively.

So, what we do know is that occupations that require a lot of forceful gripping with or without repetitive use of the wrist in a flexed or extended position seem to have the highest incidence of CTS. What about using computers? A Danish study found that people who used a keyboard had lower pressures in their carpal tunnel.[27] In other words, the study concluded that keyboarding was *not* associated with an increased incidence of CTS, though there was an association between using a mouse and developing symptoms of CTS. This study, and another by the Mayo Clinic that also found no association between computer use and developing symptoms of CTS, have been widely reported in the media and taken as evidence that computer use doesn't cause CTS.[27, 28] A careful analysis of each study reveals several concerns that prevent the careful reader from agreeing with the generalizability of their conclusions. While we still don't have established evidence showing a true cause-and-effect relationship between keyboard use and developing symptoms of CTS, these widely reported studies also do not prove the absence of a relationship between keyboarding and CTS. In fact, the Danish study did show an association between symptoms and use of a mouse for more than 20 hours per week.

> **Generalizability** — The concept that the results of a study using a sample of the population can be thought of as representing the results you would observe if you studied the whole population from which the sample was drawn. This is an important concept in science because if you have a flawed study based on a sample, you cannot then apply those results to everybody.

According to the Washington State Department of Labor and Industries' Medical Treatment Guidelines for Work-Related Carpal Tunnel Syndrome Diagnosis and Treatment, for CTS to be work-related it must have three characteristics: (1) Exposure (a specific activity in the workplace causes or contributes to CTS); (2) Outcome (the diagnostic criteria for CTS must be met); and (3) Relationship (the assignment of a greater than 50% probability that the exposure caused the outcome based on generally accepted scientific evidence).[29]

The American Academy of Orthopedic Surgeons, in conjunction with the American Society for Surgery of the Hand, published a Clinical Practice Guideline (CPG) on the management of CTS that evaluated the evidence for various risk factors that have been associated with CTS (see Supplement at end of chapter for more information about CPG and for an explanation of the "star" ratings that follow).[4] They found strong evidence to support a high BMI and a high wrist or hand repetition rate at work with an increased risk of developing CTS (★ ★ ★ ★). BMI is a tool used to classify an individual's weight along a spectrum from "normal" to "overweight" to "obese" to "morbidly obese." These categories are used in research studies to identify relative risks for developing certain diseases. The measure itself is imperfect because weight as an absolute measure can be misleading. For example, are the five pounds that make you "overweight" due to extra fat or additional muscle? The difference is profound, but the BMI as constructed cannot distinguish between the two situations.

Wrist or hand repetition rate refers to what you are doing with your hands, how you are doing it, and how intensely you are doing it. If you don't have adequate time to rest your hands, if your activity involves a lot of forceful gripping and you do it repeatedly, you are at higher risk for developing CTS.

What other things may, or may not, be associated with a risk of developing CTS? There was moderate evidence to support an increased risk of developing CTS and being peri-menopausal; your specific wrist ratio or wrist index (a measure of the ratio of how thick your wrist is compared to how wide it is); having rheumatoid arthritis; psychosocial factors; having upper extremity tendonopathies nearer the hand; gardening; increased hand activity above a certain threshold (ACGIH Hand Activity Level); assembly-line work; computer work; exposure of the hand and wrist to vibration; tendonitis; and workplace forceful grip or exertion (★ ★ ★).[4] Finally, there was limited evidence to support being on dialysis, having fibromyalgia, varicosities, or a

> **Tendonopathies**—A general term that refers to disorders affecting tendons, including acute injury (from overuse) and chronic injury that is not healed. These disorders can occur anywhere along the tendon but are most common where the tendon originates and where the tendon inserts.

distal radius fracture (broken bone) with an increased risk of developing (★ ★).[4]

Moderate evidence suggests that increased physical activity is associated with a lower risk of developing CTS (★ ★ ★) and that there is no associated risk of developing CTS and the use of oral contraception or female hormone replacement therapy (★ ★ ★).[4] There is limited evidence to show that race, ethnicity, or level of education for a female are associated with either an increased or decreased risk of developing CTS (★ ★).[4]

When the CPG group looked at the relationship between specific factors and the development of CTS, they found conflicting results supported by limited evidence for diabetes, age, gender, genetics, comorbid drug use, smoking, wrist bending, and workplace type (★★).[4] The available evidence did not point to any consistent relationship.

And what about the relationship between CTS and work? While there is no established cause-and-effect relationship between work activities and CTS, the bottom line is that there does appear to be a strong association among workers in certain occupations. These individuals often spend much of their workday operating in environments that are not ergonomically optimized for their individual needs. It is the continual, forceful repetitive use of the wrist and hands without correct positioning that may be most important, highlighting the importance of proper ergonomics when performing activities. What is more difficult to understand is the extent to which the individual's own physiology may be contributing to the development of CTS. In other words, there are many other conditions associated with CTS, and it is possible individuals may be predisposed to developing CTS when employed in occupations that place greater stress on the median nerve. Other individuals may tolerate these occupations without developing any symptoms of CTS.

The lack of clarity that results from the best evidence

Ergonomic environment—refers to the space in which you work and how it is set up in relation to your body. It includes the equipment you use, how it is used (for example, repetitive or prolonged use), and how your body is positioned during that use. These all contribute to increasing the efficiency and comfort of your working environment.

complicates decisions about whether CTS is a work-related condition in any one individual's circumstance. If you have opened a workmen's compensation claim for CTS, you may be frustrated that it wasn't accepted or that they are contesting your claim. "How can that be? My hands are numb!" you say. Hopefully, the previous discussion will help you understand why your worker's compensation insurance may be asking for more information or even contesting your claim. As you can see, while you may have no doubt that your hands are numb and tingling, it is harder to determine what is responsible. This leads to a lot of confusion, added stress to you, and added cost to the healthcare system.

SUPPLEMENT

AAOS/ASSH CLINICAL PRACTICE GUIDELINES

The American Academy of Orthopaedic Surgeons, in concert with the American Society for Surgery of the Hand, produced a clinical practice guideline (CPG) for the diagnosis and management of CTS. The full text of the CPG can be found at www.aaos.org/ctsguideline. We will discuss the recommendations in the sections on diagnosis and treatment.

What is a "clinical practice guideline" (CPG)? It is a collection of recommendations regarding the diagnosis and treatment of a condition.

Who writes the CPG? The CPG is produced by a working group whose participants are physicians and researchers with extensive experience treating the condition in question. The working group requires individuals who can translate research findings into clinical practice and interpret the quality of the research produced. This is an important task for the working group, evaluating the quality of the evidence upon which the recommendations are based. For the CTS CPG, the two major professional organizations that represent orthopedic and hand surgery have collaborated to develop the CPG. They are the American Academy of Orthopedic Surgeons and the American Society for Surgery of the Hand.

What conditions have CPGs? Certain medical conditions have been selected for CPGs, based on their overall impact on society. It is a laborious process to produce a CPG: it requires a significant investment on the part of the members of the working group to review literature, formulate recommendations, and negotiate their acceptance. Because of the work involved, not all conditions have CPGs. Examples of other CPG produced by the AAOS include Achilles tendon rupture, anterior cruciate ligament (ACL) injuries, distal radius (wrist) fractures, shoulder joint arthritis, hip fractures in the elderly, arthritis of the knee, rotator cuff problems, and spinal compression fractures.

How are CPGs used in everyday practice? Providers can review their practice pattern in the context of the CPG. One benefit of the CPG is to provide practitioners with the benefit of a comprehensive review that they, themselves, do not have the resources to perform. Providers can evaluate their individual practice and, when it differs from the CPG, evaluate the CPG recommendation and determine if they need to change practice behavior. CPGs are not, however, cookie-cutter templates that relegate the practice of medicine to a robotic algorithm that obviates the need for human interaction.

What is the result produced by a CPG? The product of a CPG is a series of recommendations regarding the clinical condition addressed by the CPG. The CPG can focus on the diagnosis, treatment, or both for a specific clinical condition. The recommendations are presented in summary form but require the reader to consider the full body of evidence, as the recommendations are carefully worded to reflect the limited conclusions one can draw from the available evidence.

Recommendations in a CPG are reported by their relative strength, based on the available evidence. According to the AAOS/ASSH Clinical Practice Guideline on the Management of Carpal Tunnel Syndrome, the following descriptions define their strength of recommendations:[4]

- **Strong** (overall strength of evidence is strong) recommendations have evidence from two or more high quality studies, with consistent findings for recommending for or against the intervention. Strong recommendations have a four-star rating (★ ★ ★ ★).
- **Moderate** (overall strength of evidence is moderate) recommendations have evidence from two or more moderate

quality studies with consistent findings, or evidence from a single high-quality study, recommending for or against the intervention. Moderate recommendations have a three-star (out of four) visual rating (★ ★ ★).

Ͼ **Limited** (overall strength of evidence is low strength or conflicting) recommendations have evidence from two or more low quality studies with consistent findings or evidence from a single moderate quality study recommending for or against the intervention or diagnostic test, or the evidence is insufficient or conflicting and does not allow a recommendation for or against the intervention. Limited recommendations have a two-star (out of four) visual rating (★ ★).

Ͼ **Consensus** (overall, there is no evidence) recommendations do not have any supporting evidence. In the absence of reliable evidence, the guideline development group is making a recommendation based on their clinical opinions. Consensus statements are published in a separate, complementary document and not the formal CPG. Consensus recommendations have a one-star (out of four) visual rating (★).

Chapter 3 Summary

- At any point in time, it is estimated that between 3% and 8% of the population has CTS.

- Certain occupations have a higher prevalence, ranging from 17% to 61%. These occupations tend to involve forceful repetitive hand motions in non-neutral wrist positions. Examples of such occupations: butchers, grinders, grocery-store workers, frozen-food factory workers, etc.

- CTS appears to become more common as we age, with an estimated 82% of cases occurring in patients over 40 years old.

- Females represent 65% to 75% of cases.

- 60% to 70% of CTS cases occur in both hands.

- The cost of care for patients with active workmen's compensation claims costs is *three times* the cost of care provided to workers without an active workmen's compensation claim and *five times* the cost of treating non-workers.

- The AAOS/ASSH Clinical Practice Guideline (CPG) on the management of CTS identified various risk factors that have been associated with CTS.

4

WHAT HAPPENS IF I HAVE CARPAL TUNNEL SYNDROME?

How a disease or condition develops untreated in a patient over time is referred to as its "natural history." If you have CTS, its natural history may follow one of several paths. Sometimes, the symptoms occur after a brief period of intensive activity and resolve spontaneously after stopping the activity. In this setting, if the offending activity is avoided, the symptoms may never recur. Pregnancy is another example of an isolated circumstance, after which the symptoms may resolve and never return. Included in this scenario are poor ergonomic environments and poorly managed medical conditions that once corrected can eliminate the symptoms and prevent their recurrence.

In other cases, compression of the median nerve may result from repeated activities that produce pressure in the carpal tunnel that is simply greater than what the individual's body can tolerate.

Still others will begin to develop symptoms of CTS without any identifiable cause, so-called idiopathic CTS.

If the symptoms of CTS do not resolve and are left untreated, one path that the natural history can take is disease progression. The numbness becomes more frequent, occurs more easily with any activity, and persists almost constantly. Eventually, the nerve supply to muscles is affected, resulting in hand weakness. In the case of CTS, there is a nerve branch that supplies the abductor pollicis brevis muscle, which branches off the median nerve just after it exits the carpal tunnel. When this nerve is affected by CTS, the muscle it supplies undergoes atrophy (see figure 13).

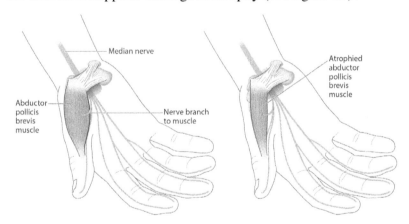

Figure 13
Thumb Muscle Atrophy
As CTS progresses, the muscles supplied by the nerve are compromised and can lose their ability to function. The resulting muscle atrophy, causing weakness and difficulty with everyday tasks like buttoning a shirt, may never recover after treatment.

The goal of any nerve surgery, and what defines successful surgery, is to stop the progression of symptoms by relieving the pressure on the nerve—successful nerve surgery just stops the condition where it is. After the nerve pressure has been relieved, it is up to nature and your intrinsic healing potential to restore the nerve function and reinnervate the muscle. Unfortunately, once the atrophy has set in it is difficult to recover muscle bulk and strength, despite adequate surgical treatment. Again, all surgery does is relieve the pressure on the nerve; pressure that was causing the muscle input from the nerve to decrease. If the pressure continues over a long enough period, it is possible that the nerve may not be able to regain its ability to supply the muscle. The challenge for us is we do not know when that point in time will occur, thus the emphasis on reversing symptoms whether by nonoperative or operative treatment.

Because of the numbness, patients also complain of the loss of dexterity, difficulty with fine motor tasks (buttoning a dress shirt) and dropping things. The loss of sensation is subtle at first but as CTS progresses you can lose the ability to feel objects that you are holding in your hand. If the nerve is not working properly, your brain has no way of knowing how much pressure to apply because it isn't getting any feedback. When this happens, if you aren't looking at the object visually to give your brain information about how much pressure to apply, gravity will simply pull the object from your hand. This is the fate of many a favorite coffee cup or glass, which is frustrating to no end for patients.

Pain can also be present from the hand and wrist, all the way up to the shoulder. Though pain is not a primary symptom with CTS, many patients do describe experiencing what they call pain. Often, they will feel an "electrical-like" shock that starts at the wrist and either shoots into the fingers or up the forearm. Forceful gripping can also cause this "pain" that patients describe. Every so often, I will have a patient tell me that after surgery for CTS their shoulder pain went away! Yes, in some cases, the pressure on the nerve can cause discomfort that even reaches the shoulder. This is explained by the path of the nerve as it travels from the hand up the forearm, arm and across the shoulder up into the neck. The afferent signal (sensory information related to the pinched nerve) is transmitted to the brain and the nerve is irritated along its entire path.

As the condition advances, there does come a point along the progression of CTS when the symptoms become irreversible. At this point, even after surgical treatment, the numbness doesn't change, and the atrophied muscles do not rebuild themselves. We do not have a way to tell exactly when that will happen, but it is a risk that increases the longer the condition exists. It is important to treat CTS symptoms and prevent their progression. Early intervention has the best chance of minimizing the long-term risk of damage.

All nerves that supply muscle make their connection to muscle using a structure called the motor endplate, which converts the nerve impulse into muscle activity. After 12 to 18 months without any nerve supply (as can be the case with severe CTS), the motor endplates are resorbed and disappear. Even if you could re-establish a nerve supply, there is nothing at the other end for the nerve to make a connection with to make the muscle work (see figure 14). This may help explain why at some point, even with surgical treatment, the symptoms of CTS cannot be reversed. At this point, surgery may help relieve some of the persistent tingling and may improve pain, but it cannot bring back the muscles or restore the sensation.

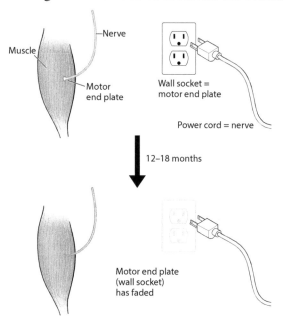

Figure 14
Loss of Nerve-to-Muscle Communication
When the median nerve is compromised in CTS, it cannot supply the muscles it innervates. An important part of the nerve-to-muscle communication is the motor endplate and after about 12 to 18 months without adequate nerve supply, the motor endplates are resorbed by the body. This is the case with chronic carpal tunnel syndrome where the abductor pollicis brevis muscle loses its nerve supply over time and the muscle atrophies. Even if you can restore the nerve supply (by releasing the carpal tunnel), the muscle cannot accept the nerve input because the motor endplates have disappeared.

Treatments, both operative and nonoperative, are designed to intervene and alter the natural history. By taking proactive steps to reverse the condition, the pressure on the median nerve can be relieved before any of the damage becomes permanent. That is why it is important to recognize the symptoms, accurately make the diagnosis, and take the necessary steps to eliminate symptoms and prevent their recurrence.

The next section describes in detail the symptoms of CTS, how the diagnosis is made (including what tests are used), and what other conditions can be confused with CTS. This discussion will help you understand what is happening and improve the quality of any interaction with your healthcare provider.

Chapter 4 Summary

- The natural history of CTS ultimately takes one of two paths: regression (it goes away); or progression (it gets worse).

- If the muscle supplied by the median nerve (abductor pollicis brevis) loses its nerve supply, it can atrophy causing weakness and difficulty with fine motor skills.

- Once atrophy sets in, it may never recover, even with successful treatment of CTS

- After 12 to 18 months without any nerve supply (as can happen with chronic CTS), the motor endplates are resorbed by the body. Then, even if you can restore nerve supply by releasing the nerve, there is nothing for the nerve to connect to at the muscle.

- Treatments, both operative and nonoperative, are designed to intervene and alter the natural history. By taking proactive steps to reverse the condition, the pressure on the median nerve can be relieved before any of the damage becomes permanent.

SECTION II

HOW DO I KNOW IF I HAVE CARPAL TUNNEL SYNDROME?

HOW IS CARPAL TUNNEL SYNDROME DIAGNOSED?

T he hallmark of CTS is numbness and tingling in the hand and
wrist along the path supplied by the median nerve (see figure
15). Pain may also be present and occur in the same general

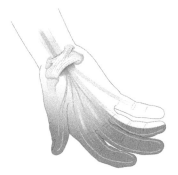

Figure 15
Sensory Distribution of the Median Nerve
The median nerve is responsible for sensation to the thumb, index, middle,
and ½ of the ring finger (shaded area).

distribution as the numbness. Because the nerve is like a two-lane
highway that sends messages in both directions, patients will often

describe electrical shocks that shoot up and down the arm and forearm (see figure 16). Though less common, people can also experience pain on the small finger side of the hand, forearm, arm, and even the shoulder because of carpal tunnel syndrome.

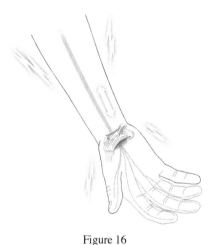

Figure 16
Electrical Shocks and CTS
Patients often describe "electrical shocks" that shoot up and down the arm and hand. These sensations are produced by pressure on the median nerve, and their paths follow the course of the median nerve in the arm and hand.

These symptoms usually go away with treatment of the carpal tunnel syndrome. However, this does not mean that if you have arm or shoulder pain then you have carpal tunnel syndrome. Often patients experiencing symptoms of carpal tunnel syndrome will unknowingly alter the use of their hand, and this can place abnormal stresses on other parts of the limb. As the sensation in your fingers decreases, you will increase the force needed to grip objects because you are no longer matching force to feedback. You are, in a sense, over-matching the force used to make sure you accomplish the task (holding a glass, turning a screw or gripping an object). The force mismatch can increase the stress on the tendinous origin of your wrist extensors (or flexors) resulting in degeneration and dysfunction. When the wrist extensors are dysfunctional, we call this condition lateral elbow pain, also known as lateral epicondylitis or "tennis elbow," and it is often present in people with carpal tunnel syndrome. When the wrist flexors are dysfunctional, we call this condition medial elbow pain, also known as medial epicondylitis, or "golfer's elbow". Symptoms of lateral elbow pain can sometimes be an important clue to the presence of early carpal tunnel syndrome.

The first question you will likely be asked is which what part of your hand is numb? An important piece of information that patients are often not aware of is which part of the hand is affected. Because CTS produces symptoms in a defined area of the hand, this is important information that helps to differentiate CTS from other conditions. It is perfectly understandable that patients sometimes don't know which part of their hand is tingling. You have come to the office because your hand is numb or tingling and just want it fixed! Paying attention to the parts of your hand that are tingling and being able to describe it is an important part of making the diagnosis of CTS. Remember, the median nerve supplies a specific area of the hand (see figure 15). Because of the anatomy, the fingers affected are generally the thumb, index, middle, and ½ of the ring finger (the side next to the middle finger). Furthermore, the tingling is only on the palm side of the hand. Tingling that involves the small finger or the back of the hand may suggest an alternative diagnosis. Taking the time to notice which part of your hand is affected and when the symptoms occur will make the visit with your healthcare provider more efficient and speed the time to an accurate diagnosis.

When a patient presents with signs and symptoms suggestive of CTS, we begin with a thorough history and listen to their description of the symptoms, the most common of which are listed in Table 5.

TABLE 5
Carpal Tunnel Symptoms

↻ Numbness or tingling in the hand (index, middle and ring fingers)

↻ Nighttime presence of numbness and tingling

↻ Pain in the wrist with activity

↻ Electrical-like shock sensations into the hand or up the forearm

↻ Loss of feeling in the fingers that results in difficulty with fine-motor activity

---

Aside from the numbness, patients will often describe tingling in the hand at night. This so-called "nighttime numbness and tingling" is another hallmark of CTS. However, it is important to distinguish this from occasional numbness that can occur if you are sleeping on your arm. Patients will often notice that symptoms become worse when performing certain activities: driving a car, talking on the phone, reading a book, or preparing their hair. These activities provoke symptoms because they all place the wrist in a position of either flexion or extension while force is applied. This increases the pressure on the median nerve within the carpal tunnel, causing symptoms to increase.

Patients will also describe what we call the "flick test," in which they will flick or shake their hand to relieve the tingling (see figure 17). Other symptoms that patients report with less frequency include cramping of the hand or fingers with or without activity, fatigue with use of the hand, cold intolerance, and shoulder or forearm pain.

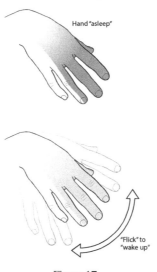

Figure 17
Flick Test
Illustration of the "flick test" wherein patients who start to feel numbness and tingling will shake their hand as shown, in an attempt they will often say, to restore blood flow

to their hand. Whatever the effect, patients do say that this flicking motion seems to temporarily relieve their symptoms.

Sometimes the symptoms begin to occur when there has been a change in activity, and other times the symptoms seem to occur out of the blue. For example, moving to a new computer workstation that is not set up properly can result in a lot of extremity discomfort and coincide with the onset of symptoms, as can a sudden increase in the amount of repetitive work done with the hands. Symptoms can also occur during pregnancy or simply begin without any identifiable event.

After we listen to the patient's story, the likely diagnosis or diagnoses often becomes clear, and the next step is to ask directed questions and perform a physical exam to both confirm our diagnosis and rule out other potential causes of numbness and tingling in the hand. You can think of this process as one of hypothesis formulation (listening

Hypothesis—an idea, or proposed explanation, developed based on limited information that explains an observation and serves as the starting point for further investigation. In medicine, your description of symptoms (observation) is the limited information we use to develop an hypothesis, which we further test with ad-ditional questions and a physical examination (investigation).

to your story) and then testing (asking specific questions and performing a physical exam). With experience, this process happens very fast and is almost undetectable by an observer unless they know what to look for in the healthcare provider-patient interaction. Some questions your healthcare provider might ask are shown in Table 6.

TABLE 6
Questions Your Doctor Might Ask You about Your Symptoms

⌐ Do you wake up at night with your hand numb or tingling?

⌐ Do your symptoms get worse with activity (for example: driving a car, reading a book, talking on the phone, fixing your hair)?

⌐ Do you have neck pain?

⌐ Do you feel electrical-like sensations coming from your neck that shoot down into your hand?

⌐ Do you feel electrical-like sensations starting at or around your wrist?

⌐ Do your feet tingle too?

⌐ How do you relieve the symptoms—do you shake or flick your hand?

These questions are designed to evaluate other potential conditions and make sure that the story told by the patient matches the diagnosis of CTS. Sometimes what may sound like CTS turns out to be another condition, such as a herniated disk in the neck

or generalized nerve dysfunction (peripheral neuropathy). Table 7
shows other conditions that can be confused with CTS.

TABLE 7
Conditions That May Look like Carpal Tunnel Syndrome

- Peripheral neuropathy (idiopathic, chemotherapy-associated)
- Cervical spine disk herniation
- Diabetic neuropathy
- Thoracic outlet syndrome
- Wrist flexor tenosynovitis or tendonitis
- Wrist arthritis (including thumb carpometacarpal joint arthritis)
- Hypothyroidism
- Raynaud's phenomenon or disease
- Arterial injury or thrombosis
- Nerve laceration
- Neuroma
- Brachial plexus injury
- Other nerve entrapment syndromes
- Pain syndromes

There are several surveys or questionnaires that you may be
asked to complete. A list of some of these is shown in Table 8.

TABLE 8
Common Carpal Tunnel Syndrome Questionnaires and Surveys

ℭ Boston Carpal Tunnel Questionnaire

ℭ DASH (Disabilities of the arm, shoulder, and hand)

ℭ MHQ (Michigan Hand Outcomes Questionnaire)

ℭ PEM (Patient Evaluation Measures)

ℭ SF-12 or SF-36 Short Form Health Survey

These are all designed, in one way or another, to help with making the diagnosis of CTS. Many of these are used in academic studies, and they generally have been shown to have reasonable validity (that is, they measure what they intend to measure). Because it is labor intensive to administer and track these questionnaires, they are not used as often in private practice. Most healthcare providers will incorporate a few select questions they find useful into their discussion with the patient; however, the surveys are not a necessary condition for making the diagnosis of CTS.

Validity—Tells us how well a test measures what it is intended to measure.

History—The process by which a doctor gathers information from you about your condition and what has been happening up until the time of your visit.

Because the first step in evaluating a patient involves taking a history, it is helpful to know what parts of the history may suggest CTS. All healthcare providers will have their preferred diagnostic pathway they follow when taking a history. Table 9 shows parts of the patient history that, in isolation, do not show any relationship to the presence of CTS when diagnosed by an electrodiagnostic study (more about this test later).[4] This means that as far as the evidence shows, the answers to any of the questions in Table 9, when considered independently, are not helpful in determining if you have CTS (★ ★ ★).[4]

TABLE 9
Patient History Items Not Related to the Presence of CTS
ℭ Your gender
ℭ Your ethnicity
ℭ If you have symptoms in both hands
ℭ If you have diabetes
ℭ If your symptoms are worse at night
ℭ How long you have been having symptoms
ℭ Where you feel your symptoms along your hand and arm
ℭ Whether you are right- or left-handed
ℭ Age
ℭ Your body mass index (just because it is high doesn't mean you have CTS and vice-versa)

Patients who report frequent numbness and tingling do appear to have a greater chance of having CTS, but the opposite cannot be said with a high degree of certainty based on the available evidence (★ ★ ★).[4]

In addition to asking patients questions about their risk factors, activities, other medical conditions, etc., part of the history also involves listening for when patients describe what we think are physical signs associated with CTS. One common sign is what we call the "flick test" (where a patient shakes or flicks the affected hand to relieve the tingling sensation) (see figure 17). While it certainly seems that CTS is common in patients who describe this sign, the evidence cannot definitively establish using it *alone* as a reliable marker for ruling in or ruling out CTS (★ ★ ★ ★).[4]

Another physical sign commonly associated with CTS is atrophy of the thumb muscle supplied by the median nerve (APB, abductor pollicis brevis muscle) (see figure 18). This occurs when the pressure on the nerve progresses to the point where it disrupts the ability of the nerve to supply muscles. The APB muscle gets its supply from a branch of the median nerve that exits right after the carpal tunnel, so it is thought to be a sensitive indicator of pressure on the median nerve in the carpal tunnel. According to the CTS clinical practice guideline, there is strong evidence (★ ★ ★ ★) for using atrophy of the APB muscle to rule in CTS, but its absence cannot be relied upon to rule out CTS.[4]

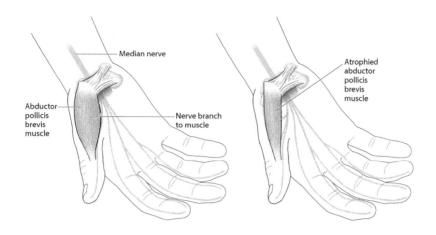

Figure 18
Thenar Muscle Atrophy
A branch of the median nerve (recurrent motor branch) exits the end of the carpal tunnel
and supplies the abductor pollicis brevis muscle. When CTS progress, this nerve branch
is affected and loses its ability to supply the muscle—leading to wasting and atrophy.

After listening to the patient and asking questions, the next step is to examine the patient in the context of the signs and symptoms. For CTS, there are a few physical exam tests that in the past have been thought to be suggestive of the diagnosis. The best evidence suggests that, in isolation, none of them can stand alone as a reliable determinant for making the diagnosis of CTS (★ ★ ★).[4] Some are better than others, and the highest yield appears to be when one or more is used in combination, which improves the sensitivity and specificity

Sensitivity—Refers to the ability of a test to correctly identify someone who has the condition the test is supposed to identify (a true positive).

Specificity—Refers to the ability of a test to correctly identify those who do not have the condition the test is supposed to identify (a true negative).

for making the diagnosis. (In other words, when combined, the tests best identify the condition when the tests are positive and exclude the condition when the tests are negative.) The bottom line, however, is that there is currently no one single test that both defines a patient as having the diagnosis of CTS and excludes the patient who does not have CTS.

TABLE 10
Common Physical Exam Tests for Carpal Tunnel Syndrome

 Special tests: Phalen's test, Tinel's test, Durkan compression test, reverse Phalen's test, CTS-relief maneuver, tethered median nerve test.

 Sensory tests: Semmes-Weinstein monofilament testing, 2-point discrimination, vibrometry testing, tuning fork, pin prick sensory deficit.

 Motor tests: Manual motor testing of thenar muscles (thenar weakness or thumb abduction weakness).

Table 10 shows some of the physical exam tests used to diagnose CTS. There is no perfect physical exam test that defines CTS. There is some evidence that combining one or more tests can increase the sensitivity and specificity of the diagnosis. In practical terms, however, the history is often most revealing and the only physical exam test that I rely on is the Durkan compression test. All of the other tests have a combined sensitivity and specificity that is too low to be of any real use in the clinic. This is where the real world meets the academic world and while different tests are fun to study and write papers about, the diagnosis of CTS for an experienced examiner is primarily based on the patient's history and symptoms with the physical exam being used to rule out other possible diagnoses as opposed to ruling in the diagnosis of CTS.

Testing of sensation can be helpful, but it is important to recognize that the condition is advanced if there are true sensory deficits. Altered sensation, as identified by vibrometry (the ability to sense vibration), is thought to be the earliest sign of CTS. Vibration testing is cumbersome to perform and, therefore, not routinely performed in the office setting (see figure 19). Semmes-Weinstein monofilament testing is more likely to be performed in the office and

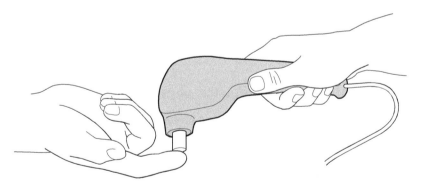

Figure 19
Vibrometry Testing
When assessing for early nerve dysfunction, vibrometry is a sensitive test for detecting carpal tunnel syndrome. Because it is cumbersome, it is not commonly used in the clinical setting.

can detect altered light touch sensation attributable to CTS (see figure 20). Finally, your doctor may test your ability to discriminate two points at the tip of your finger (see figure 21). Two-point discrimination only becomes abnormal when the condition is advanced.

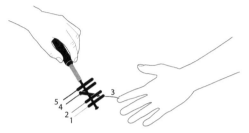

With nerve damage, patient can't feel #1 or #2

Figure 20
Semmes-Weinstein Monofilament Testing
Semmes-Weinstein monofilament testing is a common method used to assess sensation in the clinical setting. This will often be one of the first sensory tests to show an abnormality as symptoms of CTS progress.

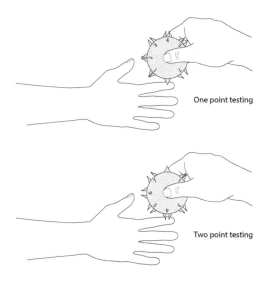

One point testing

Two point testing

Figure 21
Two-Point Discrimination
Two-point discrimination testing is another common method of testing sensation in the clinical setting. This test will be the last of the sensory tests to show an abnormality and when it does, the symptoms of CTS are often severe.

After arriving at the diagnosis of CTS, at some point along your course of treatment, your healthcare provider may recommend an electrodiagnostic test, or nerve conduction study (NCS). A NCS can consist of two parts: a study of the nerve conduction velocity (NCV) and a study of the nerve supply to the muscle, electromyography (EMG). We refer to the test as either a NCS or an NCV/EMG.

The NCV portion of the test measures the ability of your nerve to conduct an impulse over a fixed distance (see figure 22). When the distance over which the nerve is tested includes the carpal and the conduction is slow, we consider this to be consistent with the diagnosis of CTS. It is important to know that CTS, however, is first and foremost a clinical diagnosis. The NCV test can provide some helpful information about the severity of the condition, other nerves that may be affected (in the case of a disk herniation in the neck or peripheral neuropathy).

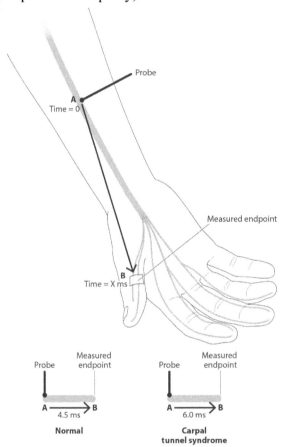

Figure 22
Nerve Conduction Testing for CTS
A nerve conduction velocity test (NCV) attempts to measure the nerve's ability to conduct an impulse over a fixed distance. The nerve is stimulated at point "A" and then the machine measures how long it takes the impulse to travel to point "B." When the nerve is under pressure, as is the case with CTS, the impulse will take longer to go from point "A" to point "B." How long it takes can be used as a measure of severity and can help guide clinical decision-making. The NCV test is also useful because if the median

nerve conduction across the carpal tunnel is not slowed, it can suggest the need to search elsewhere for the source of the symptoms.

The EMG test portion of a NCS evaluates to what degree the muscles supplied by the nerve in question have been damaged (for the median nerve, this is the abductor pollicis brevis, APB). There are many ways a muscles can act in response to altered simulation by a nerve and some of the different types of responses evaluated during the test are: (1) how the muscle responds to a needle being inserted into it (it should not have any measurable reaction); (2) how the muscle recruits additional muscle fibers in response to stimulation (it should gradually "ask for more help" by recruiting more fibers as the stimulus increases); and (3) does it show signs of chronic denervation (changes in how the muscle fiber responds when it has been "sick" for a long time). The APB muscle receives its nerve supply from a branch of the median nerve that arises just beyond the carpal tunnel. When the condition is severe, the nerve supply to the APB is lost. We call this acute denervation of the muscle and surgery is recommended (see figure 23).

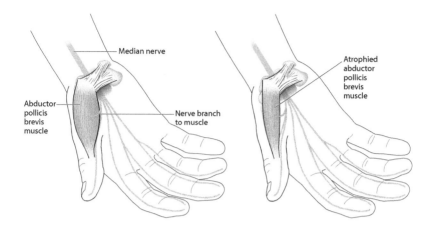

Figure 23
Loss of Thumb Muscle Nerve Supply with Severe CTS
When CTS progresses, an important thumb muscle can lose its nerve supply and waste away. When the EMG test picks up the acute (sudden) loss of nerve supply to this muscle, surgery is recommended to minimize irreversible loss of muscle function.

When there is a workmen's compensation claim associated with CTS, a NCS is often mandated by the insurance company as a requirement to establish the diagnosis. However, one can have a "normal" NCS and still have CTS. We call this "electrodiagnostically negative" CTS, and in this instance a diagnostic injection can be helpful (more about this later).

The NCV test is probably the most commonly used diagnostic test for CTS, and the easiest way to think about it is that it is a test that measures how fast your nerves can transmit an impulse over a fixed distance. The nerve is evaluated over multiple fixed-distance segments in the extremity, and the time it takes for the nerve impulse to get from the start (point A) to the end (point B) of the segment is recorded. When it takes longer for the impulse to get from point A to point B, we interpret that as meaning the nerve has a problem with conduction (which is one possible result of pressure on a nerve). When the nerve impulse moves normally everywhere within the extremity and then slows down only for the segment where the carpal tunnel is between point A and point B, then we interpret that to mean that the patient has CTS.

As mentioned above, sometimes patients will have the signs and symptoms of CTS but have a normal NCS; this is called "electrodiagnostically negative CTS." This occurs in fewer than 10% of patients who have clinical signs and symptoms consistent with CTS.[30] In cases where the patient has clinical symptoms consistent with the diagnosis of CTS and a normal NCS, a steroid injection can be helpful in the treatment pathway. When patients get good relief of their symptoms after an injection for some period of time and the symptoms return, then surgery may be considered with the expectation that it will provide a level of symptom relief like the injection.

In clinical practice, I do see patients who present with signs and symptoms of CTS and who have a negative NCS. When the clinical suspicion is high enough and there is a positive response to a steroid injection, these patients do well after undergoing surgery for CTS. This is consistent with the findings of Grundberg, who found relief in 31 of 32 hands with negative NCS (NCV/EMG) and clinical signs and symptoms of CTS.[31] However, this is not a common occurrence and requires carefully listening patients to understand the symptoms they are reporting. In everyday life, non-verbal communication is an important part of our daily interaction. Successful communication with people is dependent upon our ability to read, respond, and react to the non-verbal clues that are being offered. While this occurs somewhat intuitively over time as we develop experience in communicating, one must always carefully listen and observe to be effective with communication.

Clinical diagnosis is similar in this respect and, in the case of CTS, physician intuition (defined as confidence in the diagnosis and puzzlement with respect to patient symptoms) is a specific and accurate predictor of negative electrodiagnostic studies in patients being evaluated for possible CTS using electrodiagnostic studies.[32] You cannot rely solely on just what a patient says, you must consider the context in which they say it, allow for inaccuracy in how they define terms as they use them and consider alternative explanations that could be described similarly. It is very difficult to create an artificial construct for clinical decision-making using an algorithm that captures this non-verbal information. This highlights just how important the human patient-physician interaction is to the delivery of healthcare.

I will discuss the concept of "arm ache" in more detail later, but for now it is enough to know that the primary symptom of CTS is numbness, and when there is a strong presence of pain in the setting of mildly positive or normal NCS, other diagnoses must be considered. I do see patients who clinically look for all the world like they have CTS, have mildly positive NCS, respond appropriately to a steroid injection, and undergo surgery for CTS. Despite improvement in their symptoms, they still have persistent complaints referable to the median nerve. When considering alternative diagnoses, I often see a condition called thoracic outlet syndrome (TOS). I am fortunate to have a wonderful physiatrist in my community who is skilled at treating this condition. When I send these patients to him, they respond well to a diagnostic injection in the scalene muscle and to nonoperative treatment of TOS. Fortunately, I do not have patients who undergo surgery for CTS with negative NCS who do not meaningfully improve. While this seems to reinforce the research findings about physician intuition, it also highlights the importance of listening to patients and being aware of the presence of "arm ache" and other confounding factors.

Consideration of alternative diagnoses that might explain a patient's symptoms is a critical part of treating patients. Lo et al. found that about one-half of patients in a community practice referred for NCS to evaluate suspected CTS did not have results consistent with the diagnosis of CTS.[33] This finding highlights the importance of combining a good clinical understanding of CTS with a careful consideration of the patient's history. Interestingly, although the study was not designed to tease out the strength of the referring physician's belief in a diagnosis of CTS, they did not find any significant difference between non-specialists (family physicians, rheumatologists, physiatrists, neurologists, general surgeons, internists) and specialists when it came to the percentage of patients who did not have a diagnosis of CTS based on NCS findings. In this study, alternative diagnoses were most related to musculoskeletal conditions (tendonitis, epicondylitis, trigger finger, disk herniation in neck, myofascial pain or strain, arthritis), but notably in about one-half of the patients with normal NCS, no alternative diagnosis could be established. When no definitive diagnosis can be established, it is important to be aware of psychological factors that can affect a patient's clinical presentation. Depression, somatization, and catastrophization can all contribute to the development of "arm ache" (a non-specific complaint of pain in the limb, like a headache).

It is important to remember that despite the concept of CTS being relatively straightforward, there is still conflicting evidence when it comes to using NCS in the diagnosis of CTS. One important role of NCS is to look for evidence of other conditions that may look like CTS (generalized nerve dysfunction—peripheral neuropathy, pinched nerve in neck—cervical radiculopathy and nerve compression not located at carpal tunnel).

Technical aspects of NCS testing can also contribute to confusion. For example, the NCV test only tests the larger myelinated nerve fibers and not the smaller myelinated and unmyelinated nerve fibers.[34] We know that when the NCV is abnormal, the larger myelinated nerve fibers are demyelinated or have a loss of axons.[35] So, one explanation for the presence of CTS symptoms with a normal NCS is that the symptoms are due to dysfunction of the smaller myelinated and unmyelinated nerve fibers that are not measured by the NCV test. If there are enough healthy, large nerve fibers to conduct an impulse, the test will appear normal when the patient has signs and symptoms consistent with CTS. This is where the physician's intuition and experience treating patients with CTS is important. As has been shown by Watson et al., there is a strong correlation between physician intuition and NCS results.[32] This is the art of medicine, and it cannot be replicated by machines or computer algorithms.

Sometimes a patient will only exhibit symptoms of CTS with activity. Such "dynamic" CTS will often not show up on a NCS unless the condition progresses, or you were able to test the individual during the activity (not practical in real life).

Dhong et al. looked at 138 patients (222 hands) and found that patients who had similar levels of self-reported clinical symptom severity had a wide range of NCS findings.[36] There is a saying in medicine, "We treat patients and not test results," and this study highlights the truth in that saying. Physicians must interpret the results of a NCS in the context of the patient's clinical presentation and cannot rely on the test's absolute findings to guide treatment.

There are other tests that have been evaluated for their ability to diagnose CTS. Future research may prove the merits of magnetic resonance imaging (MRI) and ultrasound, but at present, they are used primarily in research settings and are considered investigational until they are proven to accurately establish the diagnosis of CTS. The AAOS/ASSH CPG found moderate evidence (★ ★ ★) for not routinely using MRI for the diagnosis of CTS and limited evidence (★ ★) for not routinely using ul3trasound for the diagnosis of CTS.[4] There is only limited evidence for the use of a hand-held NCV device that was introduced to the market a few years ago in the hope that it could simplify obtaining electrodiagnostic data (★ ★).[4]

Further research may identify some combination of diagnostic questionnaires and electrodiagnostic testing that provides better and more reliable diagnostic information. While the primary research limitation is the lack of a true gold standard for diagnosis, there is moderate evidence supporting the use of diagnostic questionnaires with electrodiagnostic studies to aid in the diagnosis of CTS (★ ★ ★).[4]

Chapter 5 Summary

- ℃ A hallmark of CTS is numbness and tingling in the hand and wrist along the path supplied by the median nerve.

- ℃ Nighttime numbness and tingling in the hand is another hallmark of CTS.

- ℃ CTS produces symptoms in a defined area of the hand, this is important information that helps to differentiate CTS from other conditions.

- ℃ Currently, no one test both defines which patients have the diagnosis of CTS and excludes those patients who do not have CTS.

- ℃ Often, a nerve conduction study (NCS) is recommended when the diagnosis of CTS is under consideration. It is important to know that CTS, however, is first and foremost a clinical diagnosis. The NCS can provide some helpful information about the severity of the condition, other nerves that may be affected, and to what degree the muscles have been damaged.

- ℃ The lack of a true gold standard for diagnosing CTS limits our ability to define diagnostic tests with high sensitivity and specificity.

SECTION III

TREATMENT FOR CARPAL TUNNEL SYNDROME

HOW IS CARPAL TUNNEL SYNDROME TREATED?

After establishing the correct diagnosis (a sometimes overlooked but critical detail—make sure your ladder is leaning against the correct wall before you start climbing), the next step is to act to reduce or eliminate the symptoms.

Figure 24 shows the conceptual treatment pathway after we have established the diagnosis of CTS: it is broken down into You, Your Hands, and Your Doctor. Thinking of treatment in this way empowers patients to take an active role in their treatment and well-being. The steps to be taken are relatively straightforward and the recommendations are based on the best evidence available, as outlined in the AAOS/ASSH Clinical Practice Guideline for the Treatment of Carpal Tunnel Syndrome(★★).[4]

Conceptual Treatment Pathway for Carpal Tunnel Syndrome

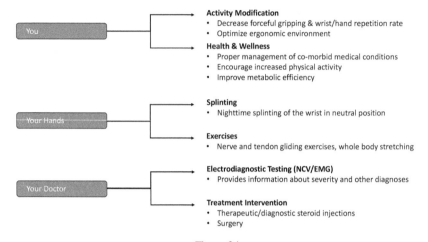

Figure 24

CTS Conceptual Treatment Pathway

Visual representation of the treatment pathway when we have established that a patient has CTS. The recommendations within the pathway are discussed in more detail in the text.

In general, we begin with a course of nonoperative treatment. There appears to be no harm in trialing nonoperative treatment for 4 to 6 weeks. If the symptoms respond to treatment and the condition improves, then we continue to manage CTS nonoperatively. If the symptoms fail to respond, then we continue down the treatment pathway until we achieve resolution of symptoms.

SPLINTING

One of the first steps we take in the treatment of CTS is to initiate splinting of the wrist at night. The splint is worn so that the wrist remains in a neutral position (see figure 25) This means that the wrist lies flat, not flexed or extended, when the splint is worn. When compared to a wrist that is flexed or extended, keeping the wrist

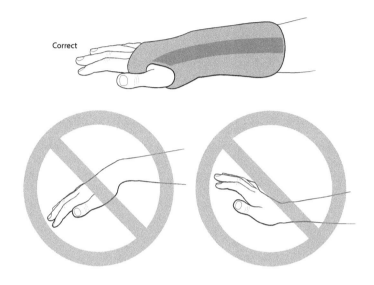

Figure 25
Using a Splint for CTS
The proper wrist position when wearing a splint for CTS is with the wrist in the neutral position. Note that the wrist is neither flexed nor extended when the splint is positioned properly. This often requires bending the metal bar along the palm side of the splint to flatten it out, so the wrist sits in the neutral position.

flat, or neutral, results in a lower pressure within the carpal tunnel. Because this is not a functional position for the wrist, the splint is only worn at night. In order to achieve a neutral wrist position, it is often necessary to modify the splint when you first get it. Out of the box, off-the-shelf splints all have a metal bar along the palm side that causes the wrist to sit extended about 15°. This is the proper anatomical position for the wrist. To get your wrist to sit in the neutral position, you will have to bend the metal bar and flatten it out until your wrist is neutral when the splint is worn. You can accomplish this either by hand or by bending the splint over the edge of a counter.

Occasionally, a splint is worn during the day when symptoms are severe. When that is the case, you can wear it in whatever position feels the most comfortable, either as it comes right out of the box or with wrist in the neutral position worn at night. AAOS/ASSH Clinical Practice Guideline for the Treatment of Carpal Tunnel Syndrome's level of evidence for splinting is strong (★ ★ ★ ★).[4]

Activity Modification

Patients will often report that certain activities will result in increased symptoms. It is important to identify any activity that is aggravating and modify or eliminate it to the greatest extent possible. The intensity or frequency of the activity can be reduced or sometimes altogether eliminated. Intensity refers to the amount of force used during an activity, while frequency refers to how often you perform the activity. Any single activity can be low intensity and high frequency, high intensity and low frequency or any combination depending upon how it is performed. Monitoring and adjusting both of these variables is important to minimizing the stress on the median nerve and resulting symptoms of CTS.

For example, if use of a keyboard is an aggravating low intensity, high-frequency activity, then using voice-activated software can reduce the keyboarding load. Taking frequent breaks can also act to diminish the frequency of the keyboarding (though it ultimately impacts overall productivity). This is where ergonomic evaluation of the workstation environments becomes important. Our bodies are not designed to sit in a single position, relatively cramped, and perform repetitive activities for eight-plus hours a day. Making sure that the ergonomic environment is optimized will reduce the stresses on the body and improve overall function. Each patient is usually able to identify aggravating activities; take the time to discover yours and work to modify them to reduce the symptoms you experience. While the AAOS/ASSH Clinical Practice Guideline for the Treatment of Carpal Tunnel Syndrome's level of evidence for activity modification is inconclusive, this may simply reflect the difficulty in obtaining adequate data. When discussing activity modification, we are really referring to the combination of patient-specific activities and appropriate ergonomics, which necessarily will be specific to the individual. It will be difficult, if not impossible, to design a satisfactory study when the "treatment" (activity modification) is so varied and individual. It is this limitation in the tools we have available for research that leads to the "inconclusive" label. However, what we know from experience is that when patients alter an offending activity or improve the ergonomic efficiency of their environment, this often correlates with a reduction in their symptoms.

HAND THERAPY

Another important component of the treatment of CTS is to engage a certified hand therapist. One aspect of the interaction will be instruction of nerve and tendon gliding exercises. These exercises promote blood flow in the nerve, which correlates with a reduction in symptoms.[37] Hand therapists, trained to evaluate a patient from the neck to the fingertips, are helpful in identifying areas for improvement in terms of ergonomics as well as ways to avoid developing associated conditions resulting from altered use of the extremity. For example, we frequently see patients with CTS develop lateral elbow pain (tennis elbow), as they compensate for the altered use of their hand and wrist. AAOS/ASSH Clinical Practice Guideline for the Treatment of Carpal Tunnel Syndrome's level of evidence for hand therapy considers only two components of the hand therapy experience: therapeutic ultrasound and phonophoresis (delivery of a drug through the skin) with ketoprofen, an anti-inflammatory medicine. The evidence was limited for therapeutic ultrasound (★ ★) and moderate for phonophoresis (★

★ ★).[4] Remember, the guideline refers specifically to ultrasound and phonophoresis (which are types of treatment delivered by a hand therapist) but not the entire experience interacting with a hand therapist. This is a critical distinction that is often overlooked when a blanket reference is made to "hand therapy" in the context of CTS.

MEDICINES

Non-steroidal anti-inflammatory medicines (NSAIDs) can be helpful to diminish swelling and may have an analgesic (pain-relieving) effect as well. Examples of NSAIDs include ibuprofen, Advil®, and Aleve®. Some providers use oral steroids to treat CTS; however, their potential benefit must be weighed against their potential side effects. Personally, I do not offer my patients oral steroids because of their potential side effects. Gabapentin, also known as Neurontin®, and the related medicine Lyrica® were developed to modulate nerve-mediated pain. When symptoms are severe and we are awaiting surgery, these medicines may provide some level of relief if the side effects are well tolerated. Some patients taking gabapentin complain of nausea and drowsiness that is not well tolerated. The AAOS/ASSH Clinical Practice Guideline for the Treatment of Carpal Tunnel Syndrome found moderate evidence that oral treatments (diuretics, gabapentin, astaxanthin capsules, NSAIDs, or pyroxidine) did not provide a benefit versus placebo in treating CTS (★ ★ ★).[4] They did find moderate evidence that oral steroids could improve patient reported outcomes over a short period (four weeks) versus placebo (★ ★ ★).[4] In clinical practice, the relief is most often temporary and stops when the steroids do— leaving you with only the negative effects of taking them.

LASERS

No discussion of medical treatment is complete without mentioning a laser! But seriously, there have been several high-quality studies evaluating the use of laser therapy as treatment for CTS. The evidence is limited (★ ★) that there might be some benefit versus placebo. As a result, it is not a part of routine treatment of CTS.[4] Lasers are expensive to purchase, and the owner must perform "X" number of procedures per month to justify the capital expense made to purchase the laser. This can create an incentive to run advertising in order to get enough patients to use the "laser" and cover the capital cost of purchasing it. If the benefit were strong enough, lasers would be used everywhere in the treatment of CTS. Also, the cost would drop considerably because as the volume increased, competition among manufacturers would drive down the cost of the technology much like calculators decades ago.

INJECTIONS

When symptoms are failing to respond satisfactorily to splinting, activity modification and exercises, the next step is often to discuss an injection of steroid medicine into the carpal tunnel (see figure 26) The injection has two purposes: first, it is helpful diagnostically and predicts good results from surgery if you have meaningful relief of symptoms after the injection[38]; and second, it is therapeutic and may result in resolution of your symptoms and the end of the condition for you.

In many cases, however, the relief from the injection is only temporary, lasting anywhere from a few days to a few weeks. This is usually the case when CTS has progressed in its severity.

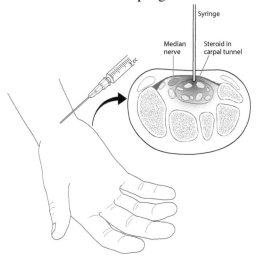

Figure 26
Injection for CTS
A steroid solution can be injected into the carpal tunnel. The fluid diffuses around the nerve and the steroid acts to decrease inflammation within the carpal tunnel. This can

be helpful to both decrease (and in some cases, eliminate) symptoms and confirm the diagnosis when symptoms are relieved, even temporarily, after the injection.

For these patients, with significant symptoms or elevated conduction delay found on electrodiagnostic studies, an injection is often only temporizing. Even when the effect is temporary, the injection can still provide valuable information and aid patients in making the decision to proceed with surgery if they are uncertain.

Another important result occasionally obtained after an injection is *no* change in symptoms. This would encourage us to explore other possible explanations for a patient's symptoms. I have many patients with a documented cervical disk herniation (in other words, a pinched nerve in the neck) and symptoms of CTS. We use the injection diagnostically in this case, and if there is good relief of symptoms, we proceed with surgery, and the patients experience much desired relief. While they may still have some residual tingling (which we attribute to the cervical disk herniation), they can relax knowing that they are not risking permanent damage to the median nerve. While there is strong evidence to support improved patient outcomes with the use of a steroid injection (★ ★ ★ ★), this effect may only be temporary as outcomes compared to those who did not receive an injection were similar after one year, despite early improvement for those who received the injection.[4] Like splinting, a local injection can be used before considering surgery.

Surgery

If the any of these steps do not provide adequate relief of a patient's symptoms of CTS, then the next step will be to discuss surgery. The fundamental principle of surgery for CTS is to divide the transverse carpal ligament (see figure 27). By doing so, the volume in the carpal tunnel is increased by about 40%, which reduces the pressure on the nerve and leads to resolution of the symptoms.

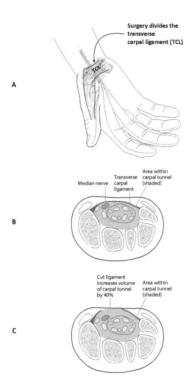

Figure 27
Dividing the Transverse Carpal Ligament
Surgery for CTS has only one objective and that is to completely divide the transverse
carpal ligament (A and B), which relieves the pressure on the median nerve as the
relative volume in the carpal tunnel increases by about 40% (C).

As we discussed earlier, if a patient waits too long to have surgery, there is the chance that the damage to the nerve will be irreversible and there will be no change in symptoms. Fortunately, this is not common, but it is important to recognize that the natural history of CTS is often one of progression, and if the symptoms are persisting, they should not be ignored. There is strong evidence (★★★★) supporting the fact that surgical release of the transverse carpal ligament should relieve symptoms and improve function in patients with CTS.[4] This is the highest level of evidence, meaning that when surgery is indicated, the evidence shows that it is an effective treatment for CTS. Further, there is strong evidence (★ ★ ★ ★) that surgical treatment of CTS should have a greater treatment benefit at 6 and 12 months, compared to splinting, NSAIDs, therapy, and a single steroid injection.[4]

There are two basic ways to perform carpal tunnel surgery: open or endoscopic (see figure 28). Your surgeon will discuss with you their preferred way for performing the surgery.

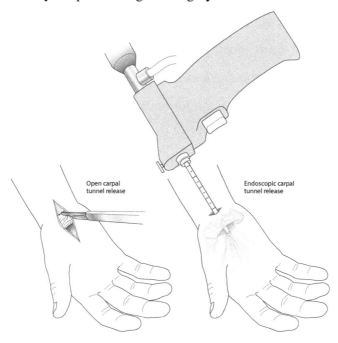

Open carpal tunnel release

Endoscopic carpal tunnel release

Figure 28
Surgical Treatment of CTS
There are two ways to treat CTS surgically, either by open or endoscopic carpal tunnel release. In each procedure, the goal is the same: divide the transverse carpal ligament.

Whether to perform a carpal tunnel release (CTR) open or endoscopically can sometimes be a source of debate within the hand surgery world, with passionate advocates for each technique. The bottom line is that while there is some evidence to suggest a quicker recovery with the endoscopic technique, the only two absolute statements that can be made are that there is a higher dollar cost in the operating room associated with the endoscopic technique and there is no established difference in clinical outcomes between open and endoscopic carpal tunnel release.[39] The AAOS/ASSH CPG for treatment of CTS found limited evidence (★ ★) that endoscopic carpal tunnel release might be favored based on possible short-term benefits.[4] I will not get into the specifics of the debate because to some extent they are irrelevant. What I will tell you is that there are some important points to keep in mind when considering surgery for CTS (or any surgery, for that matter).

First, "the surgeon-is-the-method"; this is a quote attributed to the chairman of my orthopedic department when I was a resident, and it rings true to this day. What it means is that whatever surgical technique surgeons offer a patient, it should be the one that results in the best outcomes in their hands. A surgeon who is not familiar with an endoscopic technique should not be trying to use it for surgery. Surgeons should select the operation that they are the best at performing. No matter what technique is recommended, patients need to make sure that the surgeon is comfortable and experienced with that technique. Unfortunately, there is no magic number that defines competence with a surgery. As a rule, any hand surgeon should be able to perform an open carpal tunnel release without difficulty. Endoscopic techniques require additional training and experience. Surgeons who perform all their primary, non-traumatic carpal tunnel releases endoscopically with a low conversion-to-open rate are likely committed to the technique and having climbed the learning curve, are comfortable that this is the best surgery in their hands.

I mentioned in the last paragraph a "low conversion-to-open rate"—what does this mean? "Conversion-to-open" means that at some point during a surgery, the endoscopic surgery is stopped and an open CTR is performed. The reported rate of conversion from endoscopic to open CTR in the literature is approximately 2%.[28, 40] The rate will never be zero, and for good reason. While the anatomy of the median nerve in and around the carpal tunnel is generally consistent, there are known anatomical variants that can render impossible the ability to perform a CTR endoscopically. Most commonly, there is a branch of the median nerve that exits through the roof of the carpal tunnel, and this exit point can be in the path of the knife when releasing the transverse carpal ligament. When the anatomy is not clear, it is safer to stop and convert to an open procedure than risk cutting the nerve branch. A less common reason for conversion would be equipment malfunction; for example, if the endoscope was bent and could no longer pass light. Surgeons with a high conversion-to-open rate may be less comfortable with the technique and not as confident in their ability to completely release the transverse carpal ligament.

Regardless of the technique your surgeon offers, you should know that if the transverse carpal ligament is divided completely, the outcome will be essentially the same. While some studies have shown early improvement in outcomes with the endoscopic technique, by the time patients were evaluated at one year after surgery, everyone was the same. Anecdotally, in my clinical experience that extends now over 20 years, patients who have had both an open and endoscopic carpal tunnel release without hesitation prefer the endoscopic technique, but the science has not been able to demonstrate this in an indisputable fashion. Again, the surgeon is the method, and my preference is for endoscopic surgery, as I find it more technically satisfying (you see directly everything that you are cutting, with the end of the endoscope becoming an extension of your finger as you gently probe the extent of the ligament), and my patients overwhelmingly prefer it to their experience with a prior open surgery.

Finally, the best evidence tells us that for surgical treatment of CTS, all you need to do is divide the transverse carpal ligament. Moderate evidence supports the statement that there is no benefit to routine inclusion of additional procedures beyond simple division of the transverse carpal ligament (★ ★ ★).[4] Examples of these additional procedures include epineurotomy, neurolysis, flexor tenosynovectomy, and lengthening or reconstructing the flexor retinaculum. Basically, these are all procedures that manipulate, modify, or alter the nerve and surrounding structures. All you need to do is divide the ligament—so keep it simple!

It is estimated that around 60% to 70% of individuals have CTS in both hands.[23] If you have CTS in both hands, should you have surgery on one hand at a time or do surgery on both hands at the same time? That is a question best answered by you and your surgeon in a shared decision-making process. It is a combination of personal preferences and logistics. We refer to this treatment as either "staged" (meaning there is some elapsed time between each surgery) or "simultaneous" (meaning that both surgeries are performed on the same day).

The primary benefit of simultaneous surgery is less absolute dollar cost, as most insurance companies will reimburse the surgeon and facility 50% of the second side for a bilateral procedure (meaning that if the same surgery is performed on left and right, the second side is discounted 50%). This discounting is done because the surgery fees include payment for *all* of the components of surgery, and at the margin, with a bilateral procedure, some of those costs are already accounted for by the first surgery code. The decrease in costs is offset by an increase in anesthesia fees, as these are billed by time, and adding the other side increases the time for surgery, as the team needs to break down the surgical theater, rotate the patient 180°, and re-prep and drape the patient before starting the other side.

Another potential benefit of simultaneous surgery is a shorter period of disability. However, this is harder to establish. A study attempting to demonstrate the economic benefit of simultaneous CTR versus staged CTR chose a time interval between surgeries of 6 weeks.[41] This is an excessive period of time between surgeries and thus skews the data when looking at economic analyses, making it harder to interpret the results. In my practice, staged surgeries are performed one week apart—enough time for patients to know and feel comfortable with the decision to have surgery on the second hand. About 70% to 80% of patients are ready to go with surgery on the other side a week later, while around 20% to 25% say that they need more time because they are having difficulty with functioning and having a second surgery would result in unacceptable disability. Finally, maybe 5% of patients or less tell me that they *don't* need the second surgery one week after the first hand had surgery because the second hand feels better! Usually, this occurs when one side is much worse than the other. I don't have a ready explanation, but as I discuss with them, the nervous system is connected and there is something about relieving the pressure on the affected side that seems to give them relief on the less affected other side. That means anywhere between 20% and 30% of patients in my practice will potentially experience an unacceptable level of disability if they have simultaneous CTR surgery. This is the essence of shared decision-making. According to the AAOS/ASSH CPG on treatment of CTS, the published literature contains limited evidence that is conflicting when evaluating simultaneous bilateral or staged endoscopic carpal tunnel release.[4]

From the patient's perspective, some increased absolute dollar cost is a fair trade-off for avoiding unacceptable disability. If you were to multiply the probability of unacceptable disability by the economic cost of that disability, I would venture a guess it would at least equal, if not far exceed, the difference in absolute dollar cost between simultaneous and staged CTR. This is difficult to prove, as the equation is complex, but the practical experience is that patients chose a staged procedure when faced with the decision and accept the increased dollar cost without reservation. From a behavioral economics perspective, this revealed behavior is important, as it expresses the total outcome for a complex decision-making process. Again, in a shared decision-making model for healthcare delivery, this results in high patient satisfaction.

Chapter 6 Summary

- A conceptual treatment pathway after establishing the diagnosis of CTS begins with you, and then progresses to your hands and, finally, to your doctor.

- The mainstay of CTS treatment is nonoperative: neutral night splinting, nerve and tendon gliding exercises, as well as activity modification.

- Steroid injections can be used when other nonoperative measures fail to provide adequate relief.

- Surgery is a proven treatment for CTS, with strong evidence supporting the fact that surgical release of the transverse carpal ligament should relieve symptoms and improve function in patients with CTS.

- Surgery can be done either open or endoscopically.

- Your surgeon should select the method of surgery that provides the best results in their hands. In other words, the operation that they perform the best.

SURGERY FOR CARPAL TUNNEL SYNDROME

What Happens Before Surgery

So, you have decided to undergo surgery to treat your CTS; what happens now? The first step is an office visit with your surgeon to complete the necessary paperwork and finalize the arrangements for surgery. At this visit, your surgeon will also discuss the nature of the surgery and answer any final questions. Often the path to surgery is one that has evolved over multiple clinic visits, and while the risks of surgery and its ability to achieve the desired outcome are discussed during these visits, the final preoperative visit is a good time to review this information and answer any last-minute questions that have arisen. After the preoperative visit, your surgery date is set, and the next step is to show up for surgery.

A more detailed discussion follows in the next section, but first there are some important details to make sure you understand about preparing for your surgery. First, the night before surgery, you will be asked to not eat or drink anything after midnight. (Your surgeon may instruct you to stop eating or drinking at a different time, depending upon when your surgery is scheduled, but the "nothing-by-mouth" rule after midnight is a common practice.) Second, while you should not eat or drink anything after midnight the night before surgery, your surgeon will instruct you regarding what medicines, if any, you may take with just a small sip of water on the morning of surgery. There are some medicines that are important to continue taking around the time of surgery (for example, beta-blockers) and some medicines that you should avoid (certain blood pressure medicines like Lisinopril, for example). Again, your surgeon will review your medications and make sure you take just the ones that are necessary and avoid the ones you don't need. And finally, the night before surgery, you should confirm that you have a responsible adult in whose care you can be discharged after surgery.

What Happens the Day of Surgery Part I:
Before the Operating Room

Surgery for CTS is done as an outpatient, which means that you will go home after surgery and do not need to stay in a hospital. Table 11 shows the general path you will follow after your arrival on the day of surgery.

TABLE 11
What Happens When You Arrive the Day of Surgery?

🐾 You will have been NPO for the specified time before surgery (usually eight hours)

🐾 Administrative check-in at the front desk

🐾 Taken to the pre-surgery holding area

🐾 Meet the pre-surgery nurse who will have you change clothes and get your IVs started

🐾 Meet your surgeon who will "sign" the site of surgery

🐾 Meet the anesthesia doctor who will review the anesthesia plan for surgery

🐾 Meet the circulating nurse who will escort you back to the operating room

You will be asked not to eat or drink anything for 8 hours before surgery. (Often to simplify, we simply tell patients to not eat or drink anything after midnight of the night before surgery.) Talk to your doctor about their specific requirements, as it is possible for patients to have clear liquids up to a few hours before surgery. However, because it can often be

NPO—Latin for "nils per os" which means "nothing by mouth." This is meant literally with respect to surgery; we do not want you to have any food or drink before surgery.

confusing for patients what constitutes a clear liquid, we often just tell patients to be NPO for 8 hours before surgery. Also, if the surgery center has a cancellation or is running ahead of schedule, you will not be able to move up the time of your surgery if you have not had adequate time after eating or drinking liquids. Because a carpal tunnel release surgery is a relatively short case, they are often moved around on the surgery schedule when there is a cancellation. There are times, however, when we would want you to drink fluids up until that last allowed time. For example, if you have had a previous surgery and your veins are difficult for starting an IV, we might ask you to drink fluids to "pump them up." Again, please check with your doctor to make sure you have adequate time before surgery if you are going to drink fluids.

So, why do we care about you being NPO if you are not going to sleep for surgery? Because we are cautious! Even though almost all Bier blocks are successful at anesthetizing the limb, there are some instances when we cannot get adequate anesthesia with the block. Less commonly, some patients become uncomfortable and cannot tolerate the tourniquet on their upper arm. In both instances, we need to be able to drift you off to sleep. If you have not been NPO, then we cannot provide a general anesthetic for your surgery. The risk is that you will aspirate ("spit-up") stomach contents, which will get into your airway. When this happens, patients can develop an aspiration pneumonia, which is a chemical pneumonitis (inflammation of the lungs) that is severe. So, we protect you by keeping you NPO.

What about any medicines you may take daily? Your doctor will review the medicines you take every day and instruct you on which ones to stop and which ones you can take with a sip of water the morning of surgery. Table 12 shows some general guidelines for medicines before surgery. Remember, talk to your doctor about your specific medicines.

TABLE 12
What to Do About Medicines You Take Every Day Before Surgery

Anti-inflammatory medicines (ibuprofen, Advil®, Aleve®, aspirin)	Stop these seven days before surgery
Blood-thinners (Coumadin, Plavix)	Stop these five to seven days before surgery (check with your prescribing doctor to see if you need a temporary medicine to "bridge" the period you are off the blood thinner, e.g., Lovenox.)
High blood pressure medicines (Lisinopril and other "prils", HCTZ)	Do not take this the morning of surgery.
Beta-blockers (metoprolol)	DO TAKE this the morning of surgery.
Insulin	Usually take half your normal maintenance dose the morning of surgery. Do not change dose of any baseline insulin that you may take via a pump (if you have one).
Metformin	Do not take for twenty-four hours before surgery.
Other medicines	Check with your doctor.

Remember to check with your doctor about any medicine that you take before surgery.

Blood-thinners and anti-inflammatory medicines are in a category we refer to as anti-coagulants (that is, they slow or prevent the blood in your body from clotting normally). This is an important concept around the time of surgery because unnecessary bleeding during or after surgery can lead to complications. It usually isn't an issue during surgery, because we use a tourniquet, but after surgery, if you bleed more than normal you could develop what we call a hematoma (collection of blood in or near the wound). A hematoma can result in more pronounced stiffness or additional scarring. The hematoma limits motion and creates an environment more prone to developing an infection. The bottom line is that we take very seriously any medicine that alters your natural ability to regulate bleeding in and around the time of surgery. There is some thought that in hand surgery, it may be okay to continue blood thinners without the need to stop them for surgery. Research into this question reveals that, while generally safe, there is evidence to suggest that continuing blood thinning medicines without stopping them before hand or wrist surgery is associated with a higher risk of developing a hematoma at the surgical wound or surgical site bleeding with certain proceedures.[42, 43] The AAOS/ASSH CPG on the treatment of CTS found only limited evidence to support the idea that a patient might continue to use aspirin without stopping it for surgery (★ ★).[4] Other anti-coagulants did not have studies of adequate quality to be considered.

Upon arrival at the hospital or surgery center, you will go through an administrative check-in process. This will involve confirmation of your identity, insurance information, and that all paperwork has been properly completed. After this, you will then wait until you are called back to the presurgery holding

> **Presurgery nurse**—The nurse who will be taking care of you before you enter the operating room. They are the first member of the surgery team you will meet on the day of surgery.

area. The presurgery holding area is where you will meet the presurgery nurse who will confirm your identity as well as the specific hand and the procedure to be performed. Next, you will change into a gown for surgery and the presurgery nurse will place the IVs used during surgery.

> **Anesthesia doctor**—The doctor who is responsible for the administration and monitoring of your anesthesia during and after surgery.

For carpal tunnel surgery, there are two: one on the non-surgical arm for the anesthesia doctor to use when administering sedating medicines, the preoperative antibiotic medicine and IV fluids; and a second one on the back of the hand having surgery. The IV on the back of the hand having surgery is used for the Bier block (described below), which is how your hand "goes to sleep" for the surgery. For carpal tunnel release surgery, we put your hand to sleep, not you! However, you can choose whatever level of sedation you would like; just let the anesthesia doctor know your preference. (Some people want to watch the screen during surgery and others want to drift off to sleep—the choice is yours.) Once your IVs have been placed and the pre-surgical checklist has been completed, you will meet briefly with your surgeon (who will mark the operative site) and the anesthesia doctor, who will review your anesthesia plan for surgery. The final member of the surgical team you will meet in the presurgery area is the circulating nurse for the operating room. This person will also confirm your identity and the surgery to be performed before escorting you back to the operating room.

Circulating nurse—The member of the surgery team who is responsible for the part of the operating room that is not sterile. They are the quarterback of the OR team, making sure everything is in its place and communicating with both the pre- and post-anesthesia care teams about the case.

What Happens the Day of Surgery Part II: In the Operating Room

Once in the operating room, you may feel a little bit like a car at the Indianapolis 500 race that has just pulled in for a pit stop. There will be a lot of buzzing around and activity but don't worry, it is all routine…for us. Figure 29 shows the players on the operating room team. After entering, you will be asked to lie down on the operating room table and the team working together will accomplish the following—likely at the same time:

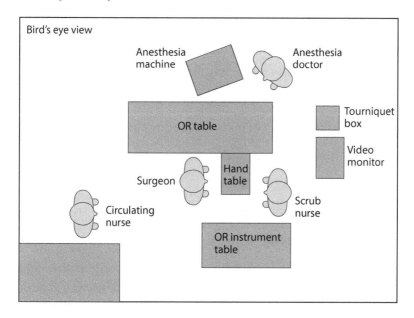

Figure 29
The Operating Room Team
Diagram showing the layout of a typical operating room and the players involved. The surgeon, who may or may not have an assistant (often an assistant is not needed for a carpal tunnel surgery), works closely with the scrub nurse throughout the case. The circulating nurse is present to help make sure all runs smooth in the OR, and the anesthesia doctor makes sure you are comfortable and pain free during your surgery.

1. The anesthesia doctor will place EKG leads on your chest and a blood pressure cuff on your non-surgical arm. They will use the IV in your non-surgical arm to deliver some sedating medicine that helps take the edge off and lets you relax.

2. Either the surgeon, surgical assistant or anesthesiologist will then place a double-bladder tourniquet on the upper part of your arm that is having surgery. First, they will apply some cotton padding called webril, followed by the tourniquet and then a sticky drape that keeps the cleaning solution off the tourniquet.

3. The circulating nurse will help either the anesthesia doctor or your surgeon with these tasks. In addition, they will cover you with a warm blanket, take your glasses, if any, and keep them safe all the while making sure you are generally comfortable.

4. The scrub nurse will be preparing the back table with the instruments used for your surgery. At this point, this is the only person in the room who has formally scrubbed and is remaining sterile.

> **Scrub nurse**—The member of the surgery team who is responsible for the instruments used during surgery. Their "back table" has all the sterile instruments, and the scrub nurse gives the instruments to the surgeon as they are needed during the surgery. They play an important role on the surgery team and, by anticipating the next step in a surgery, can make the case flow smoothly.

Once you are comfortable lying on the table and have the tourniquet in place, the Bier block procedure can begin. See figure 30 for a diagram explaining how the Bier block is performed.

Your surgeon (or the anesthesia doctor) will wrap your arm tightly with an elastic bandage called an "Eschmarch." This will squeeze most of the blood out of your veins and toward your body. When the wrap reaches the

> **Bier block**—a form of intravenous regional anesthesia that is frequently used for upper extremity surgery. It renders the affected limb numb, allowing for surgery to proceed and does not have the risks associated with general anesthesia.

tourniquet, the tourniquet bladders will be inflated and deflated sequentially (1:inflate – 2:inflate – 1:deflate) (see figure 30). At this point, the veins have been cleared of most of the blood volume and are now ready to receive the anesthetic. The anesthesia doctor will inject the IV on the back of your hand with the numbing medicine, which replaces the blood that was in your vein. Because the veins and nerves generally travel together in the limb, as the numbing medicine leaks out of the vein, it then bathes the nearby nerves and puts the arm to sleep. It is a pretty ingenious way to distribute the numbing medicine to the entire limb. The tourniquet is necessary to keep the numbing medicine from distributing throughout the body, which would dilute its effect on the limb having surgery.

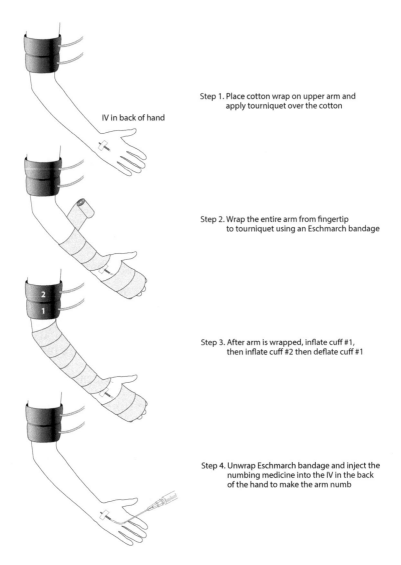

IV in back of hand

Step 1. Place cotton wrap on upper arm and apply tourniquet over the cotton

Step 2. Wrap the entire arm from fingertip to tourniquet using an Eschmarch bandage

Step 3. After arm is wrapped, inflate cuff #1, then inflate cuff #2 then deflate cuff #1

Step 4. Unwrap Eschmarch bandage and inject the numbing medicine into the IV in the back of the hand to make the arm numb

Figure 30

Bier Block for Regional Anesthesia

Surgery for CTS is commonly performed with a regional anesthesia technique called a "Bier block." The technique uses a double bladder tourniquet that restricts blood flow in the arm. That way, when the anesthesia doctor injects the IV with numbing medicine, it stays concentrated in the arm having surgery. If the tourniquet becomes uncomfortable, the anesthesia doctor can inflate the lower bladder (#1) after a few minutes, which allows for the area underneath it to become numb.

After the numbing medicine has been injected, the circulating nurse will remove the IV in the back or your hand and begin the "prep." The surgical prep, as it is called, involves cleaning the limb with a special solution that decreases the number of bacteria at the site of surgery. While this is happening, your surgeon will be outside the operating room "scrubbing" for surgery, and the anesthesia doctor will be making sure you are comfortable and completing some paperwork to make sure everything is in order.

After the arm has been cleaned, the scrub nurse will then place a series of drapes that protect and isolate your arm for surgery. They will also begin placing instruments on the table and making final preparations for surgery.

I want to take a moment to mention that the use of a Bier block is my preference based on the short duration of effect (works only when you the tourniquet is inflated) and improved patient quality of life immediately after surgery (no nausea or other problems frequently associated with general anesthesia). Some surgeons prefer general anesthesia, and others prefer to use a local anesthetic injection. There might be some geographic preference as in the literature it seems that local anesthesia may be more common in the eastern part of the United States. In Canada, it is often used out of necessity, as surgeons cannot get operating room time and have developed a way to do the surgery in their offices (so-called Wide-Awake-Local Anesthesia-No-Tourniquet, or WALANT). Your surgeon will discuss with you what is their preference; you don't want to ask them to do something that they are not experienced with or otherwise uncomfortable doing. The best evidence is limited (★ ★) to support the use of local anesthesia instead of regional anesthesia (Bier block) for carpal tunnel surgery.[4] No qualified studies were found that compare general anesthesia to either regional or local anesthesia for carpal tunnel surgery.[4] If your surgeon does choose local anesthesia, there is moderate evidence that using buffered lidocaine (instead of plain lidocaine) could result in less injection pain (★ ★ ★).[4]

Once everything is completed, the Bier block has been administered, the arm has been prepped and draped, and the surgeon is sitting at the table, you are ready for surgery to begin. Before starting, an important pause is taken for what we call the preoperative "time out" (see figure 31). The "time out" is when everyone in the room stops and makes one final check that confirms the patient's identity, procedure to be performed, the correct limb (left or right for CTR), that the correct instruments are in the room and that preoperative antibiotics have been administered. After completing the "time out," surgery is ready to begin!

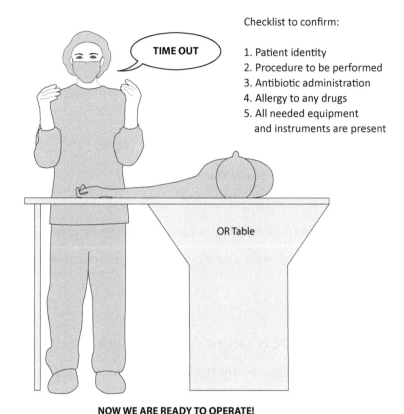

Checklist to confirm:

1. Patient identity
2. Procedure to be performed
3. Antibiotic administration
4. Allergy to any drugs
5. All needed equipment
   and instruments are present

NOW WE ARE READY TO OPERATE!

Figure 31
Preoperative Time out
The preoperative "time out" is an important step before surgery starts. It is a final "pre-flight" check when everyone in the OR stops and takes a moment to double-check what is being done and to whom.

In my practice, I administer an antibiotic before surgery to minimize the risk of a surgical site infection, and this is well supported in the published literature. Some believe that preoperative antibiotics are not necessary for carpal tunnel surgery. My personal preference is to use them based on the available literature for surgical site infections. The AAOS/ASSH CPG on the treatment of CTS found limited evidence to support the idea that there is no benefit to the routine use of prophylactic antibiotics before carpal tunnel release, because there is no demonstrated reduction in postoperative surgical site infection (★ ★).[4]

What about the Surgery Itself?

For those who have an interest (whether surgeon or patient), the basic steps involved with endoscopic carpal tunnel release are as follows:

1. Incision:
   a. Once there is adequate anesthesia (that means enough time has passed for the Bier block to set up, generally 7 to 9 minutes), an approximately one-centimeter incision is made just proximal to the major wrist crease using a 15-blade scalpel. As a rule, we try to place the incision in one of the minor wrist creases for the best cosmetic result.

2. Approach:
   a. The soft tissue is cleared over the distal forearm fascia and retinaculum, using tenotomy scissors and Ragnell retractors, to allow identification of the tendon of the palmaris longus.

b. The tendon of the palmaris longus is then retracted toward the radial (thumb) side, which protects the palmar cutaneous branch of the median nerve.

c. You have now completely exposed the distal forearm fascia where it blends into the retinaculum and can use a tenotomy scissor to penetrate the fascia. The ulnar (small finger) side Ragnell is placed at the distal (far) end of the wound to retract the tissue and fully expose the retinaculum.

d. In a stepwise manner, the retinaculum is elevated with the tenotomy scissor and divided with the scalpel. The median nerve is located directly below the retinaculum and, therefore, is being protected by the tenotomy scissor.

e. After adequately dividing the retinaculum, a narrow double-pronged skin hook is then used to keep it in an elevated position for the remainder of the procedure. The approach to the carpal tunnel has been completed, and the surgeon now has unfettered access to the carpal tunnel.

3. Inserting the Endoscope:

a. Before inserting the endoscope, the carpal tunnel must be "prepared." A synovial elevator (spoon-shaped instrument with a flat surface facing toward the carpal ligament and rounded surface facing the nerve) is used to clear soft tissue from the underside of the transverse carpal ligament. The anatomy of the transverse carpal ligament results in fibers running from left to right, or perpendicular, to the direction of the synovial elevator and produces a tactile sensation, as if you were running something across a washboard.

b. The synovial elevator is followed by sequential dilation using two dilators of increasing size.

c. After dilation, the carpal tunnel is ready for insertion of the endoscope.

4. Identifying the Distal Transverse Carpal Ligament:

a. Before dividing the ligament, it is important to identify its distal-most limit. This is readily identified by the visualization of yellow subcutaneous fat and palpation with the opposite hand index finger in the palm to demonstrate where the ligament ends (you can see this from the endoscopic view).

b. The surgeon is now ready to elevate the blade and begin dividing the ligament. The blade assembly has a U-shape and when it is pressed up against the undersurface of the transverse carpal ligament, the walls of the "U" keep the nerve protected. The blade then rises toward the top to divide the ligament when the device is engaged.

5. Dividing the Transverse Carpal Ligament:
   a. The distal portion of the ligament is divided first and will usually require multiple passes with the device to completely divide the ligament. This is a crucial step where the surgeon uses the end of the blade assembly as a "finger" to feel for any remaining transverse fibers of the ligament. The combination of direct visualization of the fibers via the endoscope and the tactile feedback as the end of the scope encounters fibers running from left to right ensures that there is a complete division of the distal fibers of the ligament.
   b. After dividing the distal portion, then the remaining proximal portion of the ligament is divided in a similar manner. At all times, when subsequent passes are made to divide the ligament, the endoscopic device is kept up within the previously cut leaves of the ligament. This important step keeps the median nerve and its common digital branches protected.
   c. Before dividing the proximal-most part of the ligament, the double-pronged skin hook is removed from the ligament and placed at the level of the skin. This step

both allows for complete division of the proximal portion and protects the skin from an inadvertent cut that results in a T-shaped incision. If it happens, the wound still has acceptable healing: avoiding the "T" is a matter of attention to detail and a desire for perfection on the part of the surgeon.

d. After completely dividing the transverse carpal ligament, the carpal tunnel is inspected using a Ragnell retractor to elevate the skin and a Freer Elevator to "feel" for any remaining fibers running left to right. This is just a careful double-check of what has been seen endoscopically. If the surgeon felt there were still any remaining transverse fibers, the endoscope can be inserted to divide the fibers.

6. Dividing the Forearm Fascia:

a. Before the transverse carpal ligament is divided, there is often a lot of pressure on the nerve (after all, if there wasn't, there probably would not be any symptoms) and after it is divided, the nerve tends to "float" up toward the skin. As this happens, the nerve can become pinched by the forearm fascia in the distal forearm.

b. To prevent such a problem, using a tenotomy scissor and Ragnell retractor, the distal three centimeters of the forearm fascia is divided under direct visualization.

One can see where the stout fascia fades and becomes thin and soft thus no longer a threat to pinch the nerve.

7. Wound Closure:

    a. The wound is now irrigated with normal saline and closed using a subcuticular 4-0 Prolene suture (placed beneath the skin level) that is removed one week after surgery.

    b. 10 cc of 0.25% Marcaine with epinephrine is injected for additional postoperative pain relief.

    c. The wound is then dressed with steri-strips, xeroform gauze, a 2 × 2 gauze dressing, webril cotton, and an ace wrap. An ace wrap is all that is necessary; no splints are needed after carpal tunnel surgery, and the AAOS/ ASSH CPG on the treatment of CTS found strong evidence to support the fact that there is no benefit to routine postoperative immobilization after carpal tunnel release (★ ★ ★ ★).[4]

8. The Surgery is Finished:

    a. The surgical drapes are then removed, and the patient is taken to the PACU (post anesthesia care unit) to recover before going home.

What Happens the Day of Surgery Part III:
After the Operating Room

The First Hour after Surgery

After the surgical procedure is completed, you will be moved to a place called the "Recovery Room" or "Post anesthesia Care Unit" (PACU). Here, depending upon your level of sedation and type of anesthesia, you will be monitored one-to-one by a nurse. The PACU is divided into two phases: Phase 1 and Phase 2. If you have a regional anesthetic (like a Bier block), you will go straight to Phase 2 after your surgery. If you have a general anesthetic (i.e., you go to sleep for your surgery), you will usually start in Phase I after your surgery where you are more closely monitored as you awaken from anesthesia. Once you are ready, you will be moved from Phase 1 to Phase 2 of the PACU. As time passes, and the effects of the various anesthesia drugs wear off, you will be offered something to drink and a light snack. Your family members will also be brought back now to sit with you in Phase 2 while you are recovering. When your vital signs are stable, your pain is well controlled, and you are tolerating a light snack, you will be cleared for discharge to home. For patients who undergo CTR surgery with a Bier block, this process all happens in about 30 to 45 minutes. If I perform two CTR surgeries back-to-back, the first patient has usually been discharged before we enter the PACU with the second patient.

When You Go Home

After meeting the same-day surgery criteria for discharge, you will be driven home by a responsible family member or friend. We recommend that you do not operate machinery or motor vehicles for the first 24 hours after surgery. You should also not make any important decisions, financial or otherwise, during this period. Once at home, you should relax and elevate the hand that had surgery. We recommend elevating between 12" and 18" above the level of your heart. Any higher and your body must work too hard to pump blood to your hand. It is important to wiggle the fingers, as this also helps to remove fluid that contributes to swelling.

What Happens After Surgery & Your Recovery

What to Expect the First 24 hours after Surgery

The hand that underwent surgery will have a light dressing consisting of a cotton wrap and an ace wrap (see figure 32). You may get some swelling beyond the end of the dressing, and this is common. However, the wrap should not feel too tight. If it does, you are welcome to loosen it to the point where it feels comfortable. The incision will be on the bottom (or palm side) of your hand at the level of the wrist and is covered with a small Vaseline gauze and a 2" square cotton pad. Try not to disturb this if you can while loosening the back side of the dressing. If your hand continues to have pain or feels too tight even after loosening the dressing, contact your surgeon immediately.

Your surgeon will likely have injected some numbing medicine at the completion of the procedure so you may have increased numbness in the hand when you go home after surgery. This numbness should wear off sometime over the next 24 hours. If your symptoms were severe before surgery, sometimes the numbness you had preoperatively can take weeks or months to improve. After surgery, in most cases, the tingling that you felt before surgery (and that may have been waking you up at night) is gone but sometimes it gets worse temporarily before getting better. Many patients get their first full night of sleep right after surgery because the hand is no longer tingling at night!

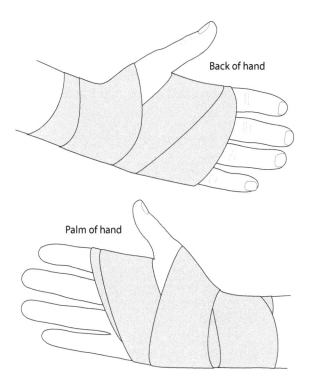

Figure 32
Postoperative Dressing
After carpal tunnel surgery, the wrist is covered with a light ace wrap dressing. Underneath the ace wrap is a cotton wrap, and beneath that is a 2 × 2 gauze sponge and a small Vaseline-covered dressing right over the wound.

The first day after surgery, if you try to use your hand for lifting or gripping activities, you may notice a phenomenon we call "pillar pain": a sharp discomfort at the base of your hand when you try to pinch or grip (see figure 33). This occurs in almost everybody after surgery, and its degree of significance varies according to the individual. Some people have very little trouble. I have had surgeons operating one week after CTR, patients go deep-sea fishing, and many others for whom the impact is minimal, whereas other folks have difficulty putting on a bra or buttoning their pants. It is not something to be worried about, and I find that simply being aware of it

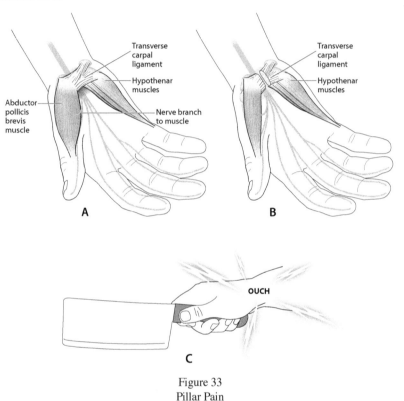

Figure 33
Pillar Pain
After dividing the transverse carpal ligament, the muscles that help move the thumb and small finger rays and take origin from the ligament lose their stable base. When this happens, patients experience pain across the palm of the hand with gripping activities. This generally resolves over time but can be a frustrating part of the early recovery period for some patients.

reduces any anxiety and seems to minimize its impact. Most research studies show that grip strength will be equal to the opposite hand (if that hand is normal) by approximately 12 weeks after surgery and that the grip strength will continue to improve for up to one year after surgery.

Many of my patients tell me that by 4 to 6 weeks after surgery, things feel great, the tingling is gone, and it just feels like a deep bruise if they push off using the palm of their hand.

After surgery, there are no formal restrictions with respect to the use of your hand, rather let pain or discomfort be your guide. Having said that, I do not recommend heavy lifting or gripping for the first 4 to 6 weeks after surgery. You will not "undo" or otherwise reverse the surgery by using your hand too much. You will, however, lead to swelling, and that can slow down your recovery.

The First Few Days after Surgery

The first few days after surgery, your focus should be on keeping the swelling down and avoiding aggravating activities. If you can tolerate anti-inflammatory medicines (like ibuprofen or Aleve®), you may use them for both pain relief and to help reduce swelling. You will have been given a prescription for pain medicine at the time of your discharge after surgery. Many patients find they need only a few pills for a couple of days. This is confirmed by a recent study that found patients took, on average, approximately five pain pills after surgery for carpal tunnel syndrome.[44] In general, the surgery is well tolerated in terms of pain. Many of my patients are able to manage their discomfort after surgery with only Tylenol® and anti-inflammatory medicines.

On the third day after surgery, you will remove the postoperative dressing and place a Band-Aid® over the wound. Up until this point in time, you have been required to keep the dressing clean and dry. You may now let shower water run over the wound and simply pat the wound dry when you are done. However, do not let your wound soak in any water (e.g., dishwater, bath water, or a hot tub) for 3 weeks after surgery. Prolonged submersion of the wound under water can cause it to soak open and let in bacteria that cause infection.

Your First Postoperative Check-Up

Approximately one week after surgery, you will return to see your surgeon for your first postoperative visit. At this appointment, your wound will be checked for signs of infection and the suture, or sutures, removed. Any questions you may now have are answered, and the next step in your recovery is reviewed. It is at this point in the recovery period that patients in my practice benefit from visiting with a hand therapist for instruction in scar massage and to review the nerve and tendon gliding exercises. Everyone is different, and some patients are ready to go after a single visit with the hand therapist, while others require more visits to optimize their recovery. In the end, you will be your own best therapist (meaning that after proper instruction, it is the work you do on your own that will benefit you the most), but I find that at least one visit with the hand therapist is the most efficient way to ensure every patient has the optimal outcome and no one falls through the cracks.

The AAOS/ASSH CPG on the treatment of carpal tunnel syndrome found moderate evidence to suggest that there is no additional benefit to routine supervised hand therapy over home programs in the immediate postoperative period. But there was no evidence meeting inclusion criteria for evaluation that compared the potential benefit of exercise versus no exercise (★ ★ ★).[4] This is consistent with my decades of clinical practice experience where each person is treated as an individual. Some patients will need only a visit or two and have excellent follow through with instruction and a home program. Others will not need to engage directed therapy at all because they remember their program from when the other hand had surgery. For these people, their outcome is not affected by attendance at hand therapy. However, other patients are reluctant to move, fearful of pain, and unsure what to do. These patients benefit from interacting with a hand therapist after surgery to maximize their outcome. The four studies evaluated in the AAOS/ASSH CPG on the treatment of CTS were focused on certain aspects of therapy, such as lasers (which we do not use), sensory re-education (the nerve will recover on its own), therapist-supervised exercises versus only at-home exercises (if you are doing the exercises, the outcome should be the same), and a ten-day therapist-supervised program versus an at-home program. The studies were only of moderate quality, with incomplete information about important parameters, which makes it difficult to draw firm conclusions.[4]

I think that it is important to take a moment and reinforce the importance of your aftercare following CTR. The condition can return, though not commonly, and if it does (assuming the surgery was performed correctly the first time), the cause is usually scarring around the nerve. This is where the nerve and tendon glides and your diligence in performing them become important. You can decrease the chances of the nerve scarring by performing the exercises that help it to glide freely within the carpal tunnel.

The Next Few Weeks after Surgery

This is the period in which you will realize the most rapid increase in the use and strength of your hand. Formal strengthening in most postoperative protocols begins at about 3 to 4 weeks after surgery (starting with light strengthening and progressing from there). Table 13 shows a standard postoperative rehabilitation protocol for after CTR surgery.

TABLE 13
Postoperative Rehabilitation after CTR Surgery

0–1 week after surgery	Light use of the hand as tolerated is allowed. No heavy lift or grip. Stop any activity if you experience pain.
1–6 weeks after surgery	Formal hand therapy begins with wound care plus tendon and nerve gliding exercises. As progress allows, light strengthening is started around week 3 to 4.
6–12 weeks after surgery	Return to full work activities is expected. Depending upon progress, you may require additional time for strengthening or for resolution of pillar pain that may limit certain activities.
12 weeks to 1 year	Some residual discomfort is not uncommon and usually goes away over the next few months. Grip strength should be about equal to the other side at 12 weeks, and you will continue improve for up to a year after surgery. Residual numbness in the fingers can also take months or more to resolve.
Work restrictions (if needed depending upon the specific job demands) up to 6 weeks after surgery.	No lift > 3 lbs. and no repetitive use of the affected extremity.

Your tingling should mostly be gone and, other than some weakness, your hand will often feel like a new hand compared to before surgery. Your activity level will be limited only by your pain level, and you can resume all activities on an "as tolerated" basis.

Most of my patients will say that by a few weeks after surgery all is well, and it just feels like a deep bruise in the palm of their hand if they try to push off with the heel of their hand. This sensation usually disappears between 4 and 6 months after surgery. Remember, however, that true numbness associated with carpal tunnel syndrome takes a long time to come on and can take a long time to get better after surgery. Even though the nerve has been decompressed, it may take months for the sensation to reach its maximum recovery.

What about Return to Work or Sport?

The short answer is as soon as you feel you are able. What this means is as your recovery progresses, you can perform any activity as soon as you are ready. There is no established timetable that applies to everybody. I have had surgeons operate one week after releasing their carpal tunnel, patients go deep-sea fishing, and even go on a trail clearing expedition three weeks after surgery.

So, what should you expect? In general, most studies show that it takes about 3 months for the grip strength to equal that of the other hand (assuming it is uninjured and did not also have a carpal tunnel release) and continues to improve for up to one year after surgery. If you can control the pace and intensity of your activities, you can return to work as soon as you like. Many of my patients will elect to have their carpal tunnel release on a Wednesday and then return to work the following Monday. As a rule, I will offer my patients time off from work until I see them back at the first postoperative visit after surgery.

For patients who have physically demanding occupations or cannot control the pace at which they will be working, I will place formal work restrictions after surgery. Patients get an individualized program based upon their unique circumstances. The restrictions can range from no work at all (for mechanics and those performing heavy manual labor) to limits on lifting (no more than 3 pounds) and repetitive use (none, in general) for up to 6 weeks after surgery. At any point in time, the restrictions can be lifted if the patient is ready.

Can Carpal Tunnel Syndrome Come Back?

It is not common, but carpal tunnel syndrome can come back. If it does recur, it is often years after the original surgery, and the mechanism causing symptoms is different. In primary carpal tunnel syndrome, the nerve is basically being pinched in the carpal tunnel. That is why releasing the carpal tunnel relieves the symptoms:

the nerve is no longer pinched. When carpal tunnel syndrome recurs, however, the mechanism is usually scarring around the nerve. The result of the scarring is to tether the nerve and prevent it from gliding when the wrist moves in flexion and extension. The tethering produces a traction-neuropraxia (nerve injury) from the constant tension on the nerve. If surgery is performed again, it is done with an open technique that allows the surgeon to remove all the scar surrounding the nerve and allow it to once again glide freely in the carpal tunnel. The postoperative program of tendon and nerve glides along with scar massage is your best means of minimizing the chances of carpal tunnel syndrome coming back.

Is Surgery the Only Answer? What about Other Treatments like Lasers, Pulse Lights, Supplements, etc.?

Without a proper scientific evaluation, we cannot know if the treatment is responsible for the observed effect. It is possible that the person taking a "special seaweed extract" also started wearing a splint, or changed their work environment or workload and voilà, the symptoms got better. If we don't properly isolate the intended treatment, we cannot know if it is responsible for the observed effect. You could easily assume that the "special seaweed extract" was the cause of symptom improvement in the example above without a rigorous scientific analysis—all you need to do now is buy some full-page, four-color newspaper advertising and you have the next greatest treatment for CTS! Only to find out later that it doesn't really work when someone critically evaluates it— but nobody comes to take back the money you made selling the "special seaweed extract".

Even with the best scientific design, research is hard to do, and it can be difficult to demonstrate relatively small responses to treatment—we refer to this as the statistical power of a study to detect a difference of a certain size. A related concept is that of a "clinically meaningful difference." In other words, it is one thing to show that the symptoms of CTS got better with a treatment, but you really want to know how much they improved and what impact that had on the patient. While showing a 5% reduction in symptoms might garner a podium presentation at a meeting or a nice publication, if that doesn't meaningfully impact the clinical course of the disease and the patient's function, then it doesn't much matter.

The AAOS/ASSH Clinical Practice Guideline has reviewed all the available evidence for both the diagnosis and treatment of CTS. This was an exhaustive undertaking that sought to place the weight of scientific evidence behind recommended treatments. Beyond what is recommended, there is simply no conclusive evidence for the successful treatment of CTS. Despite the lack of conclusive evidence, there are still proponents of various treatments, and sometimes their enthusiasm leads them to suggest their one way is the only way, and that there may be a conspiracy or bias on the part of organized medicine against their favorite treatment.

I can guarantee you, having spent time in the academic environment as a researcher and author, that any laser, light frequency, seaweed extract, or "special therapy program" that could be shown to successfully treat CTS would be a career-making discovery. If you are the scientist who shows you can eliminate CTS without surgery, you will win awards and get promoted. This is how a career is made. My response to treatments offered on the Internet and in four-color, full-page ads in your local newspaper is to paraphrase Tom Cruise's character in Jerry Maguire: "Show me the evidence!"

SUPPLEMENT:

HAND THERAPY AFTER CARPAL TUNNEL SURGERY

After the first postoperative visit, many patients find benefit from working with a hand therapist. A postoperative pathway for rehabilitation after carpal tunnel surgery is outlined below. When trying to determine the role of hand therapy after surgery for CTS, the AAOS/ASSH CPG on the treatment of CTS determined that there was moderate evidence (★ ★ ★) that supported not using routine supervised therapy after surgery for CTS.[4] But, as they readily acknowledge, there were meaningful limitations in the studies used to form the basis of their conclusion. I have always treated each patient as an individual, and everyone has different needs when it comes to their postoperative recovery. My goal is to maximize the recovery for each specific individual patient. Some patients will only need to see the exercises once, do not tend to form scars, and can easily modify their activities during the healing phase—they will not need much hand therapy at all. Other patients are fearful of moving their hands, tend to form scars, or have physically demanding jobs—these folks may need more personalized attention and instruction to maximize their outcomes. So, at the end of the day, we don't prescribe "X" number of visits for "X" number of weeks; we tailor the postoperative interaction with hand therapy to the individual and their unique needs—this results in happy patients and the best possible outcome after surgery for CTS. The information below outlines the general progression of hand therapy after surgery for CTS.

Frequency of visits: Depends upon the specific needs of the individual. We usually start with one or two visits in the first week and then after that continue based on the individual patient's progress. If patients are doing their "homework" between visits, often only a few visits are all that is needed.

Seven to ten days after surgery: (1) Wound—scar mobilization and desensitization techniques are started and continued throughout the postoperative recovery period. Scar massage will enable you to break up the scar that is forming at your incision site. Desensitization will help you to progressively retrain your brain to accept the new signals it is receiving from the freshly operated area about the incision. (2) Range of motion exercises are started that keep your tendons gliding freely across the wrist and keep your fingers moving. Moving the fingers helps to reduce scarring and edema (swelling) in the hand. You will move each of the fingers and the tendons serving them both individually and as a unit. These exercises should be performed as a group five to ten times each four times per day.

I want to take a moment and discuss why nerve and tendon gliding exercises after carpal tunnel surgery are an important part of your recovery. Carpal tunnel can come back, and when it does, it is often due to scarring in and around the nerve. When we talk about "scarring" we are referring to adhesions that form between the nerve and tendons, literally the tendon and nerve become glued together. When this happens, the nerve cannot glide freely within the carpal tunnel. As a result, as the wrist moves through an arc of motion there is a constant pulling and stretching of the nerve that can cause injury (traction neuropraxia). When you perform the nerve and tendon gliding exercises, you minimize the risk of developing these adhesions—and reduce the risk of carpal tunnel syndrome coming back.

Three to four weeks after surgery: Depending upon resolution of edema (swelling) and comfort level, light strengthening may now begin. This progresses as tolerated through week six after surgery. These exercises should be performed four times per day for five minutes each time.

Six weeks after surgery: Return to full work activities is expected by this time. Sometimes additional modified duty is needed to allow time for more strengthening or time for pillar pain to resolve, depending upon the specific job activity. Ergonomic evaluations and adaptations should be completed and in place upon the return to work. The individual is counseled to avoid forceful repetitive use of the extremity. It is important to continue with nerve and tendon glides and an overall stretching program once back at work.

Six to twelve weeks after surgery: Progressive strengthening and increased activity with most of the work being done as a home program. Most studies show that grip strength will approximate the other unaffected hand by about twelve weeks after carpal tunnel release and improves for up to one year after surgery. Sometimes, the pillar pain will persist, or there is thickening of the scar at the base of the hand. Most of this will resolve with time. True numbness that results from CTS may take months or longer to resolve, but the tingling should be largely gone by now.

Chapter 7 Summary

- ☙ If nonoperative measures are not providing adequate relief, your doctor will have a more in-depth discussion with you about the surgical treatment of CTS.
- ☙ There is an initial preoperative visit where paperwork is completed.
- ☙ Surgery is done on an outpatient basis.
- ☙ Surgery is performed with regional anesthesia (that means your hand goes to sleep, not you).
- ☙ There is an entire team dedicated to you! In addition to your surgeon, the other team members you will meet include the anesthesiologist, circulating nurse, scrub tech, and the preop, postop and PACU nurses.
- ☙ After surgery, you will be discharged to home in about an hour.
- ☙ Your surgeon will provide detailed postoperative instructions. In general, there are no formal restrictions after surgery for CTS.
- ☙ Most studies show it takes about three months for the grip strength to equal the other unaffected hand.
- ☙ Most patients, after about a month, say it just feels like a deep bruise at the base of their hand when they push against it (that feeling goes away after four to six months).

 ↻ CTS can come back, and it is usually due to scarring around
    the nerve, and thus the importance of doing your nerve and
    tendon gliding exercises after surgery.

SECTION IV

PREVENTING CARPAL TUNNEL SYNDROME

HOW CAN CARPAL TUNNEL SYNDROME BE PREVENTED?

Now that we know what CTS is and how it is treated, an important question to ask is how can it be prevented?

There is no magic bullet to prevent CTS. Because this point is important, it is worth repeating: ***There is no magic bullet that prevents CTS.*** This means that Internet ads, flyers in the mail, and full-page ads in your local newspaper or websites promising to cure CTS with "X, Y, or Z potion, cream, a laser, or special therapy program" are designed to only benefit the person who paid for the ad. Think about it for a moment and apply a common-sense test.

For many conditions affecting the musculoskeletal system, including those that relate to overuse, a certain percentage of patients will improve on their own with no intervention at all. That is correct; if nothing is done at all, some patients will be cured. Now imagine if I invented a "magic-potion extract" to cure CTS.

If I gave it to enough patients, some would get better. I could then claim that my treatment cures CTS. Such logic fails the scientific test on multiple levels. Unfortunately, the newspaper advertising section only requires a small disclaimer to avoid running afoul of the FDA guidelines.

When we want to determine if a certain treatment has the desired effect on a condition, we apply proper scientific principles and perform a rigorous analysis that can be confirmed by independent investigators. The bar is set high for a reason, and any claim of cure must meet a standard of evidence that is agreed upon by the scientific community.

All hope is not lost, however, when it comes to the prevention of CTS. There are steps that can be taken that will minimize both your risk of developing CTS and the level of symptoms if you already have CTS. What follows is a discussion of steps you can take to minimize your risk of developing CTS and, if you already have symptoms, your risk of permanent nerve damage. Notice that none of these require you to purchase a special product (other than a basic splint), use a laser, take a magic potion, or pay for a special therapy program. See Appendix B for a description of the HandGuyMD® CTS Prevention Program.

A WORD ABOUT HAND THERAPY

What is the role of hand therapy in preventing CTS? There are many ways in which working with a hand therapist can help to prevent CTS and minimize your symptoms if you already have CTS. However, not every person needs to meet with a hand therapist.

But how do you know how to get started and where to begin in the prevention of CTS? First, you will want to look for a hand therapist with the CHT designation. CHT stands for Certified Hand Therapist and is a professional designation that is only earned after demonstrating a true commitment to the study and care of conditions affecting the upper extremity. It requires five years of clinical experience and over 4,000 hours of direct hand therapy practice.

A CHT with a special interest in ergonomics can go on to become a Certified Ergonomics Assessment Specialist (CEAS). This means that they have advanced education and a deeper, demonstrated commitment to understanding how your body interacts with its environment. A CHT/CEAS will be able to look at the tasks you perform, break them down, and help you construct an optimal work environment that will reduce stresses on your overall musculoskeletal system. This will help prevent not only CTS but also a host of other common conditions that affect the hand, wrist, elbow, arm, shoulder, and even the neck and back. A few visits with a CHT/CEAS are a worthwhile investment to take care of the machine that is your body. After all, a top-quality sports car requires careful fine-tuning to provide optimal performance, and your body is no different!

In my state (Washington), a patient can see a hand therapist for a single visit without a physician's referral. After that, your physician will need to monitor and prescribe treatment by a hand therapist. The rules may be different in your state, but a visit with a hand therapist is a good place to start if you think you have symptoms consistent with CTS. Again, for all the prevention steps we are discussing, I am not aware of any permanent harm coming from attempting these for an approximately four-week period to see if your condition improves.

So, how do we think about prevention in the context of CTS? We can view prevention of CTS as steps along a prevention "staircase" (see figure 34). This staircase is divided into three "steps": You, Your Hands and Your Outlook.

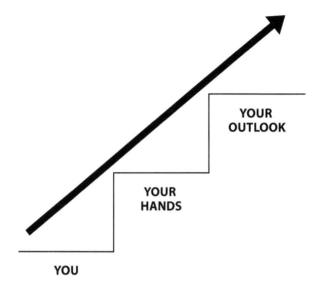

CARPAL TUNNEL PREVENTION "STAIRCASE"

Figure 34
The CTS Prevention Staircase
There are many factors that contribute to the possible prevention of CTS. One way to organize the information is to think about the many parts as an ascending staircase that progresses from You to Your Hands to Your Outlook. At each step along the way, you can act to minimize the risk of CTS development and progression.

You

The floor is simply your genetic makeup. In other words, some individuals are going to develop CTS no matter what steps are taken to prevent the condition. There is a hereditary condition which predisposes people to nerve compression syndromes like CTS. Some people have anatomical variants that put pressure on the median nerve in the carpal tunnel (for example, a low-lying finger flexor muscle belly or a smaller carpal tunnel due to the size of their bones), others grow thicker tendon linings or have masses within the carpal tunnel. You can't change your structural and genetic makeup, but by taking a proactive approach, you can help minimize symptoms and may slow the progression of the condition.

General Conditioning: Your overall level of aerobic conditioning is important to your musculoskeletal health. The benefits extend beyond simply preventing CTS—remember that there is moderate evidence that increasing physical activity and exercise is associated with a reduced risk of developing CTS (★ ★ ★).[4]

You do not need to join a fancy gym or sign up for the latest fad exercise class. Simply elevating your heartrate for a brief period is adequate. The evidence suggests that as little as thirty minutes of moderate exercise (for example, walking at a brisk pace) per day is enough to give you the maximal benefit. To understand the level of activity, "moderate exercise" essentially means that you can carry on a conversation or sing while doing it. "Vigorous intensity" exercise means you cannot converse or sing while doing the activity. You can make any activity "moderate" or "vigorous" depending upon the intensity with which you participate. And more is not necessarily better. A study in the medical journal Lancet found that the risk of experiencing key health events (all-cause mortality, diabetes, hip fracture, cardiovascular disease, coronary heart disease, stroke, depression, dementia, colon cancer, and breast cancer) all decreased with increasing moderate or vigorous physical activity up to seven hours per week.[45] After that, no further benefit was realized. So, experiment with different exercise programs and do what you find enjoyable. Further, new research shows that the benefits are cumulative and, as a result, the benefit can be realized by adding together shorter periods of exertion during the day. You do not need to get your thirty minutes all at the same time.

The US Health and Human Services Physical Activity Guidelines for Americans were updated in 2018, and the recommendations are shown in Table 14.

TABLE 14
US HHS Physical Activity Guidelines for Americans

- 150 minutes of moderate intensity physical activity per week, OR
- 75 minutes of vigorous physical activity OR
- Equivalent combination (2 minutes of moderate = 1 minute of vigorous physical activity)
- Light activity is beneficial (in individuals performing no moderate to vigorous physical activity)

For more extensive health benefits:

- 300 minutes of moderate intensity physical activity OR
- 150 minutes of vigorous physical activity OR
- Equivalent combination
- Resistance training (muscle strengthening) at least twice per week

These guidelines were originally published in 2008 and were updated for 2018.[46] The draft update, which became official in late 2018, has two important changes.[47] First, physical activity is beneficial in episodes of any length. The 2008 guidelines stated that physical activity had to come in ten-minute increments. Now, the evidence is clear that you will benefit from *any* period of activity, no matter how long it lasts. The other new recommendation is that "light activity" is beneficial if you are not performing any other physical activity (moderate or vigorous). This means that you cannot go wrong by getting moving! All you can do is help yourself in the long run by increasing your activity level today. You have heard it before—park farther away and walk, take the stairs, go for a walk in the evening, garden, or do housework with gusto. The choice is yours; our bodies were not designed to sit still all day long—just do something!

Management of Medical Conditions: CTS can be associated with many medical conditions, such as diabetes, hypothyroidism, hypertension, and obesity. If you have any of these conditions, working to bring each of these conditions under optimal control will decrease your risk of developing CTS. Checking in with your primary care doctor to make sure you have optimized the medical management of any of these conditions will benefit you beyond just your risk for developing CTS. Taking action to reduce inflammation in our bodies is a fundamental part of improving your overall health and well-being. In the context of CTS, reducing inflammation may help to prevent or reverse medical conditions that are shown to be associated with CTS. Chronic inflammation has even been associated with a risk of developing cancer. The bottom-line is that we are learning more everyday about the importance of addressing chronic inflammation and its negative consequences. Factors that contribute to low-grade, chronic inflammation in the body include a lack of proper sleep, inadequate exercise, poor management of stress and a poor diet.

Your Hands

It is at this stage where you will benefit most from acquiring the information and applying the principles outlined in this book. That is the purpose of this book: to serve as a guide to your understanding and present a comprehensive program based on evidence, not gimmicks.

What you do with your hands and how you do it can influence whether you develop CTS, or how severe your symptoms are if you already have CTS. As already mentioned, there is no established cause-and-effect relationship that can predict CTS in association with a specific activity. There are, however, strong associations between certain activities and the development of symptoms consistent with CTS. The strongest association between activity and CTS is forceful repetitive gripping with the wrist in a non-neutral position. Some examples of occupations in which this can be found are meat cutters, cable splicers, hairstylists, garment workers, assembly-line workers, mechanics, gardeners, painters, homemakers, janitors, musicians, cashiers, electronic industry workers, locksmiths, and agricultural workers (see figure 35).

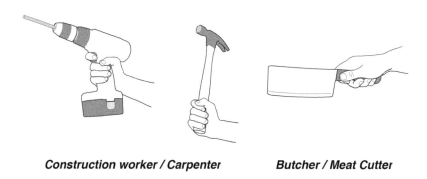

Construction worker / Carpenter   **Butcher / Meat Cutter**

Figure 35
Occupations with Increased Incidence of CTS
Workers in occupations that involve repetitive wrist motion with forceful gripping are at the highest risk for developing CTS. Some examples include construction workers, meat cutters and grocery store workers.

Splinting: If you are experiencing symptoms of CTS, start splinting your wrist at night in the neutral position. The off-the-shelf, prefabricated splint is the only "product" that has been shown to be effective. There is no "magic splint," and the only criteria is that whatever you use, it must keep your wrist flat in the neutral position, neither flexed nor extended (see figure 36).

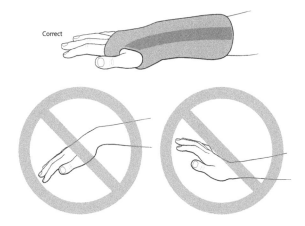

Figure 36
How to Wear a Splint for CTS
The proper wrist position when wearing a splint for CTS is with the wrist in the
neutral position. Note that the wrist is neither flexed nor extended when the splint is
positioned properly.

Nerve and Tendon Gliding Exercises: The space within the carpal tunnel is the path both the median nerve and the wrist flexor tendons follow as they enter the wrist. At this point, the nerve and tendons must glide freely as the wrist moves through an arc of motion to flex and extend. Swelling within the carpal tunnel, or simply the change in pressure as the wrist is flexed or extended, can impair the blood flow within the nerve causing the noticeable tingling. Evidence has shown that a series of nerve and tendon gliding exercises can improve blood flow to the nerve, which is associated with decreased symptoms.

Grip Force and Repetitive Use: Minimize forceful repetitive gripping with your hands. If you do need to perform repetitive gripping, try to keep your wrist neutral (which means in-line, neither flexed nor extended) as much as possible (see figure 37). Also try to take frequent breaks and minimize the time spent performing prolonged repetitive gripping with force.

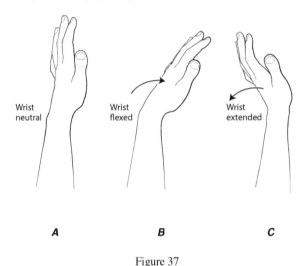

Figure 37
Wrist Position
Illustration showing wrist in (A) neutral, (B) flexed, and (C) extended positions. Forceful gripping in either the flexed or extended position while working is associated with developing symptoms of CTS.

Vibration: Limit the exposure of your hands to vibration. At work or at home, exposure to vibration, even relatively low levels of vibration, can contribute to the development of CTS symptoms. This does not mean you need to avoid mowing the lawn or blow-drying your hair. Instead, just be aware of your body, and if you start to experience symptoms suggestive of CTS, limit these activities.

Rest: Whatever you do with your hands, take frequent breaks to rest. Alternate hands and activities to avoid long periods of continuous activity. This is a critical step for many reasons. Rest allows for recovery, and recovery is a fundamental principle that is important for realizing optimal musculoskeletal health. Taking a few moments to stretch will improve blood flow to your muscles and tendons, thereby reversing the effect of any prolonged activity that requires a constant wrist or hand position. Remember, at its core, CTS is a lack of blood flow to the median nerve that results in a predictable response: tingling. Think of when you sit on your leg and it "falls asleep"; that tingling feeling you experience is essentially what is happening with CTS. When you rest, and stretch, you begin to restore blood flow to the nerve, and this reverses the symptoms that you experience. The musculoskeletal system's response to inadequate rest that doesn't allow for recovery varies by the type of tissue involved. If it is your median nerve, you get symptoms of CTS. If it is your hamstring and you overwork it, it may tear. If it's your elbow that you are continually stressing with forceful repetitive gripping, you may develop lateral elbow pain ("tennis elbow"). These rest breaks should increase your productivity at work by reducing distractions you may experience related to discomfort after prolonged activity.

Ergonomics: When trying to prevent CTS, it is important to consider what we do with our hands and how we do it. While there is no established cause-and-effect relationship, there is a strong association between CTS and activities that involve forceful repetitive gripping with the wrist in a non-neutral position (flexed or extended). Developing a better understanding of how our bodies interact with our environments and increasing the efficiency of that interaction, is an important contributor to better musculoskeletal health. Appendix B lists guidelines for the use of your hands at work and play.

The ergonomic environment in which you use your hands also has a direct impact on your function. Ergonomics can be thought of as the study of people's efficiency in their work environment. When we refer to ergonomics, in the context of carpal tunnel syndrome, we are talking about the position your body has while performing activities. For example, this means thinking about how you sit at a desk and where the objects that you need to reach for are located (keyboard, mouse, etc.). These concepts apply not only to those who sit at a desk all day, but also those who work in jobs that require the performance of repetitive tasks (cashiers, assemblers, electricians, etc.). In our discussion of ergonomic principles, it is important to remember that less than a 100% adherence to these principles does not mean you will develop upper extremity conditions. The reality is that some people can perform tasks without any difficulty, whereas others develop symptoms with only minimal activity. So, with respect to ergonomics, we want to focus on general principles that will minimize cumulative stresses.

The general principle that we want to adhere to is minimizing stress on the musculoskeletal system while you are performing repetitive tasks. Single episode events are well tolerated but repetitive activity where the musculoskeletal system is stressed will lead to problems. What does it mean for the musculoskeletal system to be "stressed"? It means that the muscles are not balanced, they are held in the same position for long periods of time, they perform the same motion over and over without adequate rest.

While the optimal ergonomic environment will necessarily be different for each person (there is no one "ergonomic way" to perform a task that applies universally), it is important to follow some general principles. Figure 38 illustrates proper body positioning while seated at a desk or computer. Some important things to note are that the major joints (hip, knee, shoulder, elbow, and ankle) are generally positioned at 90°, which reduces the tension on the muscles that move the joint. The monitor should be positioned no higher than eye level, and preferably lower, to reduce neck strain. The spine should be in a comfortable position, and you should be able to change positions frequently. Leaning back appears to be helpful in relieving stress on the low back.

A fundamental principle to remember when discussing ergonomics is that our bodies were designed for movement. That means that spending prolonged periods in fixed, static positions (such as sitting at your desk all day or performing a repeated activity for eight hours) is forcing your body to do something it naturally does not want to do. It is not surprising then, when faced with these conditions, that our bodies begin to rebel—aches, pains, muscle stiffness are all in response to our lack of movement. When we think about movement in terms of ergonomics, we want to incorporate it everywhere possible. That means in the design of workstations (sit-stand desk options, chairs that allow for comfortable repositioning throughout the day) and the structure of work (taking frequent breaks, stretching our muscles, building in exercise to the workday—for example, getting up to walk across the room to get to a filing cabinet). Bottom line: Work to incorporate movement throughout your workday!

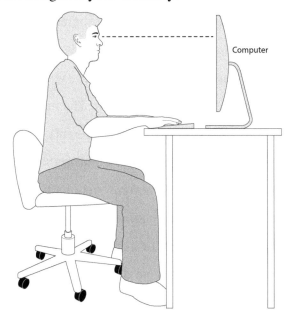

Figure 38
How to Sit at a Computer
Illustration shows the proper body position while seated at a desk or computer. Notice that the major joints (knees, hips, shoulders, elbows, and ankles) are all positioned at 90°. The spine should be in a comfortable position. The computer monitor should be no higher than eye level (and preferably lower).

Your Outlook

Your outlook, and how you approach stresses in your life, has a tremendous impact on how you feel. This can absolutely affect your body as well. The focus in medicine is often on what is going on with your body—is it broken, is something not functioning properly? A mechanic's point of view, if you will. The difference between a car and our bodies is that we have a brain that directly influences how we interact with the world. A car will simply respond to the mechanical stress you place on it during use. It does not "feel" like you are asking too much of it if you are going up hill; it does not feel pain if you keep grinding the gears when you shift or run with tires out of balance. It will simply wear out mechanically based on the laws of physics. Your body, on the other hand, has another layer of complexity that directly influences how it responds physically: your brain.

Research is demonstrating the influence of "self-efficacy" on musculoskeletal health. What does this mean? Some patients that I see in the office report symptoms suggesting a musculoskeletal disorder but do not have any specific identifiable physical exam or diagnostic findings. Such non-specific limb pain has been termed "arm ache".[48] Just like a headache or backache that can be difficult to diagnose and treat, so can arm ache. While frustrating for both the healthcare provider and the patient, improving a patient's sense of "self-efficacy" has been shown to be an effective treatment. Improving self-efficacy means encouraging a belief that you can successfully overcome your symptoms and maintain productivity in the process. It is the opposite of a "doom and gloom" outlook. The concept acknowledges that you may be experiencing some discomfort but then encourages you to look for ways to mitigate your symptoms. It is important to understand that "arm ache" is a diagnosis that applies when there is no identifiable pathophysiologic abnormality. This doesn't mean your symptoms aren't real; it just means that there is no damaging process affecting your musculoskeletal system. This means that you are free to do whatever you would like without the fear of causing more harm. This concept is often liberating for patients, providing inspiration to identify creative ways to adapt their activities. This is what we term "self-efficacy": the belief that you can overcome the obstacle and the seeking of ways to do so.

Self-efficacy—Refers to people's beliefs about their capabilities to produce specific levels of performance. It describes our confidence in our ability to exert control over our own motivation, behavior, and social environment.

When patients have a low sense of self-efficacy, we often find that they are struggling with stress at work, have an inability to adapt, or have what are termed low coping skills. While a full and complete discussion of these concepts is beyond the scope of this book, it is important to note that self-efficacy can be improved. Cognitive behavioral therapy is successful in helping patients improve their coping skills. How does this relate to CTS? Some patients who have, or think they have, CTS have pain and dysfunction in their hands and arms. When "arm ache" is the dominant contributor, they will not necessarily improve with splinting, nerve glides, or ergonomic adaptations. Your outlook, or sense of self-efficacy, is an important contributor to your musculoskeletal health! Further research has shown that this applies even for patients undergoing surgery. This concept has been given its own step on the staircase to emphasize its importance. In some ways, it can be one of the hardest things to address but it can also be one of the most important. Working on your sense of self-efficacy is a "no-lose" proposition because it will never cause us harm to have better coping skills and ways to deal with stress.

> **Cognitive Behavioral Therapy**—A type of psychotherapy in which negative patterns of thought about the self and the world are challenged to alter unwanted behavior patterns or treat a wide range of problems. It results in increased happiness by modifying dysfunctional emotions, behaviors, and thoughts.

A significant step you can take today, right now, to begin seeing the glass as being half-full is to make a decision—no matter how small. Taking a single step, making a single decision, that takes you closer to where you want to go is the first step in developing your self-efficacy.

At its core, self-efficacy is about your belief in your ability to exert some level of control over your situation. It is the belief that you can make a difference. As soon as you make a single decision that moves you in the direction you want to go, you set in motion a set of processes within your brain that create positive momentum.

In terms of how your brain functions (which is beyond the scope of this book), deciding and acting on that decision sets off a chain reaction of activity in the part of your brain that associates the positive emotions that come from a reward with the act of taking action. To be clear, it doesn't necessarily matter what activity you are performing or decision you make, it is simply that you do so. The result is that you experience a sense of being able to exert control over your situation.

Think about that for a moment; how many times have you felt overwhelmed and helpless in a situation? What happens? Are you productive or creative in finding solutions? Do you have the energy to tackle a challenging problem? When you do not feel as though you have any control over the situation, the odds are that you feel somewhat listless, unmotivated, and have difficulty finding solutions. It is not that you are not capable of doing so; it is just that for some reason you feel unmotivated. In other words, your sense of helplessness in the face of the situation results in an emotional state of apathy wherein you are not functioning at your peak ability.

What is important to know is that this is happening at the level of your brain, and the associated emotions that result are simply the result of a cause-and-effect relationship built into the design of our brain. You are not a failure or lacking in a strong-enough will to accomplish what you want. You are simply sending messages to your brain that produce an anticipated response: a lack of motivation.

Now, you can reverse this process simply by sending your brain the proper signals. That's right—as easily as you can put yourself into a "funk," you can get yourself out. The key: making a decision, taking an action that moves you in the direction you want to go—no matter how small. What happens when you do this? That same part of your brain that produces the emotional state we know as apathy (and the resulting consequences such as procrastination, listlessness, the sense that you will never succeed) sets in motion chemical reactions that produce a new state: motivation!

Your brain is, at one level, very simple (though it takes a great deal of complexity to realize this simplicity): your brain responds to pain and reward. That's basically it. So, if you make a decision or take an action that moves your closer to your desired outcome, it sets off a chain reaction in your brain that produces the emotional state known as motivation. Then, as you continue to repeat actions your brain associates with reward you will continue to feel the result (motivation). What does this mean for you? Well, when you feel motivated, you begin to see solutions where you did not see them before; you have the energy to work just a little harder at accomplishing something; you are better able to persevere when something is difficult.

Subconsciously, your brain wants to experience the feeling of reward, and you will find yourself beginning to display behaviors that will give your brain what it wants. You don't really know what is happening: you just know that now you feel energized, focused, and motivated to accomplish your goal. If you get out of the way and let your brain take over, you will move in the direction you want to go by continuing to feed your brain with the reward that it is hardwired to seek.

So, how does this relate to self-efficacy? Now imagine that you are in a work environment where you are feeling pressure to perform certain tasks. You may feel that your co-workers don't appreciate your contribution; maybe your boss doesn't seem to recognize how hard you are working. You are sitting at your desk all day, feeling the pressure mount and going home at night feeling like you are sinking in quicksand. Does that sound familiar? I would be willing to bet that if you are feeling like this, two things are happening.

First, you are not very excited about tackling the issues you face at work. Your subconscious is not working to solve the problems at hand, and you may even dread going to work. At the extreme, people turn to substances or destructive behaviors that make them "feel better," though this is always only temporary, and you never truly feel better. Such behavior can spiral into substance abuse and other destructive behaviors that destroy your life. Along the spectrum of behaviors that result from your brain's response to your interpretation of the situation are apathy, depression, forgetfulness, and a lack of excitement and creativity. Not everyone experiences every one of these, but the bottom line is most people in this state would be comfortable describing themselves as "unmotivated." Their inability to design effective strategies for resolving these stressors, and their belief that they cannot resolve them, is what we term a lack of self-efficacy.

Second, you may notice that your body hurts. Physical pain can be a manifestation of the psychological state your brain is in when you lack a sense of self-efficacy. It is difficult to establish cause and effect scientifically, but simple observation reveals this to be true. Many times, in my clinical work, I will come across patients who persist in having symptoms for which I cannot identify an anatomical cause; the so-called "arm ache" that Dr. Ring refers to in his writing. Hand surgeons see this on a regular basis, even if they can't readily identify what they are seeing.

When you take the time to ask patients about the nature of their environments, you will often find important stressors that leave them with a sense of helplessness and, you guessed it, apathy. The inability to adapt and respond constructively to the environment comes from a lack of self-efficacy. In other words, something happens at work, or at home, that increases the physiological stress your body perceives (time constraint, relationships with your co-workers or boss, workload, sense of injustice), and you begin to feel like you do not have any control over what is happening. When that feeling sets in, you are heading down the path towards apathy.

How do you stop yourself from heading down that path? You make a decision, no matter how small, that moves you in the direction you want to go. If it is a time constraint you face, maybe you decide to sit down and map out how long the task will take and what steps you need to accomplish to get it done. If it is an issue with a co-worker, maybe you decide that you are going to respond differently—if the co-worker is critical, try saying "thank you" with a smile and walking away. If you feel you are not being treated fairly, try writing down what you think would constitute fair treatment. Really, the step you take can be as large or small as you desire.

The next thing that will happen is that your brain will perceive the reward and seek to get another. You may begin to see an alternative solution; maybe you realize that if you move "X" here and push "Y" there, you can create the time you need to meet a deadline. Maybe you see an alternative strategy for dealing with your co-worker or boss. As you begin to stack up these positive events, your brain will seek more. Suddenly, you find yourself working a little later, maybe, to meet that deadline and feeling good about it. Maybe you decide to stay late tonight and then make special plans to do something another night with your kids or spouse. Now, what has happened? You are accomplishing your goal and making time for your family. Hmmm...sounds like you enjoy what you are doing. Some might call that, well, motivated. We would say you are exercising your sense of self-efficacy.

I can pretty much guarantee you that I do not see people in my office with "arm-ache" who have this outlook on life. That is how it all ties together. We can't necessarily give you a pill to magically make you "motivated," but we can prescribe an exercise that will set in motion a process that will result in your feeling motivated: make a decision and take an action that moves you positively in the direction you want to go.

So, what does all this have to do with CTS? A lot and its impact extends beyond just CTS to many conditions affecting the musculoskeletal system (various forms of "tendonitis," wrist pain, tennis elbow, shoulder pain, neck and back pain). While you certainly can have an anatomic abnormality that results in CTS, or another musculoskeletal condition, you are far less likely to have pain and dysfunction that is without an obvious anatomic abnormality if you have a strong sense of self-efficacy. I know that this section may seem a little out of place in a book about CTS, but these are important concepts that are emerging as we better understand the mind-body connection. If all you did was read this section, you will benefit in life regardless of whether you ever develop CTS.

Our ability to handle stress has a direct influence on both our bodies and our sense of self-efficacy. In fact, it is possible that a significant portion of the "arm ache" phenomenon that Dr. Ring writes about is derivative of our exposure to chronic stress.

Real, or perceived, stress results in the activation of our natural fight-or-flight response; this explains why you feel a rush of energy if you step off a curb and almost get hit by a car! When something like this happens, there is a flood of cortisol that enters our bloodstream and, via the resulting hormone cascade, you realize greater sensory acuity, strength, changes in blood flow, and the mobilization of energy stores within the body: all the good things that need to happen for your body to be ready for "fight or flight."[49] However, this system was designed to work only on the occasional basis.

Unfortunately, with our constant exposure to stress today (both physical and psychological), we are running this system at near-maximal capacity on a near-constant basis. This has detrimental consequences for both our brains and our bodies. The result of chronic exposure to stress influences a long list of health problems, including those affecting the musculoskeletal system (inflammation, tendonitis, aches, and pains) and other organ systems (diabetes, obesity, depression).[50]

Two concepts are worth discussing at this point: "catastrophizing" and focused breathing. First catastrophizing, which can be the harder concept to understand: When patients "think the worst," or "blow things out of proportion," they are said to catastrophize their symptoms. This is the idea of the glass being half-empty—back to the idea of self-efficacy that we just discussed. As you begin to see the glass as half-full, your outlook changes. Your ability to manage the situation and evaluate alternatives improves.

This is where cognitive behavioral therapy can be helpful because many of us have ingrained patterns of thinking that subconsciously lead us down the glass is half-empty path. While a full discussion is beyond the scope of this book, cognitive behavioral therapy has been shown to have a positive effect on mood, affect, and self-efficacy. This can be hard work, but the impact will go beyond your musculoskeletal health and extend to all areas of your life.

Focused breathing—A technique for mindful breathing where individuals focus their attention on their breath, from inhale to a brief hold to exhale. It makes breath the focus of concentration.

The easier concept to understand is focused breathing. There is tremendous general therapeutic value in breathing. Taking full deep breaths, as described below, delivers oxygen to our bodies, promotes good health, and improves our metabolic efficiency. If you think about it carefully, how many times during the day do you take a full, deep breath? Probably not very often. What happens when you get stressed or nervous? Your breathing becomes faster and shallower. What is the advice you hear: "Take a deep breath." What do you see athletes doing before a big shot or speakers before getting on stage? They take a deep breath. Why? Because it promotes well-being and is calming. There is a neurophysiological response to deep breathing that is immediate and impactful.

So how do you do it? One simple technique is to inhale for a count of two and hold for a count of four–eight, followed by exhaling for a count of four—a 1:2-4:1 ratio (see figure 39). This can be repeated ten times. There are other techniques that use a 4:7:8 ratio, for example. The exact ratio is not as important as the simple act of taking focused deep breaths. You can do this as often as you like during the day and for as many breaths as you find helpful. For example, if you are taking a break from keyboarding and stretching, it would also be a good time to do some deep breathing. If you find yourself feeling overwhelmed by your workload or a task, stop for a minute and take a series of deep breaths. You are likely to find that when you return to the task, you feel more positive.

Begin by breathing deeply through your nostrils to completely fill your lungs. Next, hold the breath for the desired time. (It can be difficult to hold the breath for a 4x count, but you can work up to it with practice.) Finally, slowly exhale through your mouth. Repeating the process in a controlled manner will prevent you from becoming light-headed. The deep breathing should never cause you to become light-headed or dizzy. If you are, you may be breathing too rapidly. Just slow down and focus on taking full deep breaths and gradually exhaling.

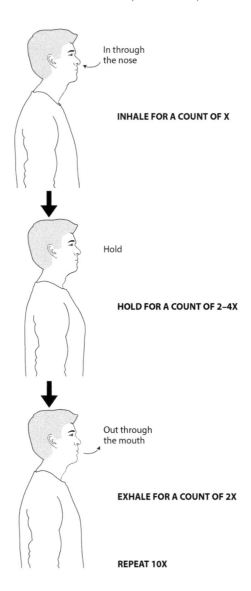

In through
the nose

INHALE FOR A COUNT OF X

Hold

HOLD FOR A COUNT OF 2–4X

Out through
the mouth

EXHALE FOR A COUNT OF 2X

REPEAT 10X

Figure 39
Deep Breathing Technique
This illustration shows one technique for deep breathing. Inhale for a count of "X," hold
for a count of 2–4 times "X," and exhale for a count of two 2 times "X." This may be
repeated as many times as you feel necessary to achieve a sense of relaxation and calm.
This is a 1:2-4:2 ratio; some advocate a 4:7:8 ratio—experiment and find what works
best for you. (Note: you should stop immediately if you become light-headed, dizzy, or
short of breath.)

So, you now have the most up to date, evidence-based information about how to prevent CTS. What you do with this information is up to you. If you do nothing, it will not help. You can only benefit if you act. Though the recommendations are sound, not everyone who follows them will avoid developing CTS. Even with strict adherence, underlying medical conditions or anatomical variations may still lead to CTS. The best that we can do is to minimize our risk and avoid creating an environment that increases the risk of developing CTS.

At this point, it is important to know that if you are experiencing symptoms consistent with CTS and have not had a reduction in your symptoms after trialing splinting, exercises and altering your work environment, then the next step should be to make an appointment with a qualified medical professional. Many people will have resolution of their symptoms after splinting only, while others find things only improve after changing their work environment. Whatever the case, I have never seen any permanent harm from trialing any or all of these recommendations for a one-month period. If, after a month, the symptoms are still present, then make an appointment with your healthcare provider. (Note: If your symptoms are progressing and getting worse, then don't wait, and make an appointment with a qualified medical professional right away.)

Chapter 8 Summary

- ℭ There is no magic bullet to prevent CTS
- ℭ CTS prevention can be conceptualized as a "staircase" progressing from You à Your Hands à Your Outlook
- ℭ **You:**
  - o Genetic makeup
  - o General aerobic conditioning
  - o Management of underlying medical conditions
  - o Reduce chronic inflammation
- ℭ **Your hands:**
  - o Splint wrist at night at first sign of symptoms
  - o Perform nerve and tendon gliding exercises along with whole body stretches
  - o Minimize forceful, repetitive gripping
  - o Limit exposure to vibration
  - o Take frequent breaks from repetitive activity to allow for rest and recovery
  - o Optimize the ergonomic environment
- ℭ **Your Outlook:**
  - o Minimize catastrophizing
  - o Increase sense of self-efficacy
  - o Improve your management of stress
  - o See the glass as "half-full"
  - o Practice mindful, focused breathing

CONCLUSION

C TS is a common condition that affects millions of Americans every day, and many more millions worldwide. It begins as more of a nuisance but then progresses to become a debilitating condition that disrupts sleep, work and everyday activities. After reading the HandGuyMD® Patient Guide: Carpal Tunnel Syndrome, you now have a thorough and up to date understanding of CTS, what it is, what it is not and what you can do if your hands are numb and tingling. Importantly, you also have evidence-based information about how it is treated and how it can be prevented.

As discussed in the book, there is no magic bullet that prevents CTS, however there are things that you can do to minimize your risk of developing CTS. Review the CTS prevention staircase and address each step: You, Your Hands, Your Outlook. See Appendix B for a concise summary and description of the HandGuyMD® CTS Prevention Program.

If your condition progresses and you enter the treatment pathway, you now understand what is being recommended and why. Appendix A presents a review of the treatment pathway for

CTS. Evaluating evidence from the AAOS/ASSH Clinical Practice Guideline on the Treatment of Carpal Tunnel Syndrome enables you to see why certain treatments are offered and others are not. As you have read, you do not need fancy devices, special lasers or potions, proprietary exercises or foods to treat CTS. The only device backed by the weight of evidence is an inexpensive wrist splint. There is also a set of standard nerve and tendon gliding exercises you can learn to perform at home. Finally, because the condition does not always respond to these initial measures, surgery may be necessary to reverse the disease process and minimize the risk of permanent nerve damage. The information in the HandGuyMD® Patient Guide: Carpal Tunnel Syndrome provides you with a thorough understanding of surgery for CTS and what to expect during your recovery.

You are to be congratulated for taking proactive steps to understand why your hands are numb and tingling. As more and more people take to the internet to search for information, it is critical that they can find reliable, trusted information—the same information and education that they would receive in a visit with their healthcare provider. This book does not replace a visit with your healthcare provider, as the missing critical piece is examining you in the context of your symptoms, but it does provide the exact same information and education that gets communicated during a visit with a hand surgery specialist.

When you consider the time lost from work, commuting to your appointment and time waiting for the actual visit, the "cost" of a visit is significant. More than the cost of the professional fee you will be billed, it is likely that you will lose a half-day of work and experience frustration at the commute and time spent waiting. Because these variables discourage people from making an appointment, ready access to reliable, trusted information about non-life-threatening conditions like CTS will improve the overall health of our population. In addition to taking steps to minimize the risk of developing CTS, applying the **HandGuyMD® SMA/RT Strategy** enables you to take early action to see if your symptoms improve. Finally, you can recognize when things are not getting better and feel good about committing your time and energy for a visit with your healthcare provider. A visit that will be much more efficient for you now that you understand not only what is troubling you but why you are presenting to the office.

Please feel free to let me know how the HandGuyMD® Patient Guide: Carpal Tunnel Syndrome has helped you, and how it can be improved from your perspective (email: DrWren@HandGuyMD.com). Visit www.HandGuyMD.com whenever you need expert help for your hands and to learn more about applying the **HandGuyMD® SMA/RT Strategy** to specific conditions using information and education about diagnosis, treatment, and prevention.

As a society, we have changed how we seek information about health-related conditions. No longer do we simply call up and schedule a visit with our healthcare provider in a few weeks. Instead, we search the internet or visit expensive Emergency Room or Urgent Care facilities, only to get a referral to yet another healthcare provider. I see this every day in my clinical practice—misinformation and confusion from internet searches and the added expense when a costly Emergency Room or Urgent Care visit is followed by still another office visit. Resources like the HandGuyMD® Patient Guide: Carpal Tunnel Syndrome, the **HandGuyMD® SMA/RT Strategy** and www.HandGuyMD.com are a model for reducing cost and improving the quality of our overall health.

Appendix A:

HANDGUYMD®
CTS TREATMENT PROGRAM

This section describes the HandGuyMD® CTS Treatment Program that has been successfully used with thousands of patients over two decades. Yes, this is the exact same information used every day in clinical practice. By reading this information you will have condensed in one place a complete description of what is recommended, why and what to expect as a result. The education and information provided by the HandGuyMD® CTS Treatment Program will improve the quality of any healthcare provider visit, increase compliance with treatment due to better comprehension while reducing stress and confusion.

Treatment for carpal tunnel syndrome progresses along a pathway that starts with the simple and moves progressively to the more complex and invasive.* In general, our goal is to get out of nature's way and give your body time to respond appropriately and eliminate the symptoms of CTS. This does not occur in everybody, however, and it is important for you to observe your response to treatment and report when you are not getting better. When symptoms do not improve after a month using a specific intervention, it is time to consider moving to the next step in treatment. If your symptoms are improving and your hands are no longer numb and tingling, then you are getting better, and you do not need to progress to the next step. Just keep doing what you are doing and if the numbness and tingling do not return, then we can consider the CTS to have gone away.

We think of treatment for CTS as consisting of many components. When the diagnosis of CTS has been established, a conceptual framework for thinking about the treatment of CTS focuses on three main areas: You, Your Hands, and Your Doctor (see figure 40). More detail about the information discussed below can be found in the relevant sections of this text (Chapters 6 and 7); the purpose of this appendix is to provide a concise summary for easy reference.

---

* *Remember, we are talking about numbness and tingling that occurs gradually over time as is the case with compressive neuropathy. Any new numbness or tingling with injury (broken bone, crushed hand, or arm, fall on the arm or hand, etc.), sudden weakness in your arm or hand, or numbness on the left side of your body (possibly including your jaw), with or without chest pain, should be evaluated immediately by a qualified medical professional to make sure there is not an emergent issue that requires immediate intervention.*

Conceptual Treatment Pathway for Carpal Tunnel Syndrome

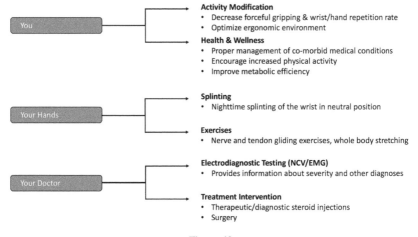

Activity Modification
- Decrease forceful gripping & wrist/hand repetition rate
- Optimize ergonomic environment

Health & Wellness
- Proper management of co-morbid medical conditions
- Encourage increased physical activity
- Improve metabolic efficiency

Splinting
- Nighttime splinting of the wrist in neutral position

Exercises
- Nerve and tendon gliding exercises, whole body stretching

Electrodiagnostic Testing (NCV/EMG)
- Provides information about severity and other diagnoses

Treatment Intervention
- Therapeutic/diagnostic steroid injections
- Surgery

Figure 40
CTS Treatment Pathway
Visual representation of the treatment pathway when we have established that a patient has CTS. The recommendations within the pathway are discussed in more detail in the text.

YOU

When thinking about You, we are focused on the proactive changes that you can make that will reduce the risk of symptom progression and, hopefully, result in a reduction of symptoms and prevent them from ever returning.

ACTIVITY MODIFICATION

One area to consider is activity modification. This means reducing the hand or wrist repetition rate, resting your hands, and making sure that your ergonomic environment is optimized to reduce tension in your musculoskeletal system.

- ℭ **Keep your wrist in a neutral position.** When performing activities, try to avoid bending your wrist for prolonged periods.
- ℭ **Use proper grip technique.** Avoid gripping with just your fingertips and try to use your whole hand. Doing so allows you to engage larger muscles and minimize pinch force, which increases the pressure on the median nerve in the carpal tunnel.
- ℭ **Minimize repetition with activities.** Avoid forceful gripping and repetitive motion for long periods. If it can't be avoided, then be sure to take frequent breaks, switch hands, alternate tasks, minimize holding objects for long periods with your hand or wrist in the same position.
- ℭ **Rest your hands.** Take frequent breaks to avoid prolonged activity without changing hand or wrist position. When you are taking a break, be sure to do some general stretching as well as nerve and tendon gliding exercises.
- ℭ **Reduce speed and force of activity.** When performing repetitive tasks, reducing both speed and force minimizes the risk of developing symptoms of CTS. You are allowing your body time to adjust to the activity and recover—think

of yourself like an athlete who knows that continuous training will not allow for the needed rest that is critical for recovery between games. The same principle applies with our bodies—it is all about rest and recovery.

Ͼ **Limit the exposure of your hands to vibration.** At work or at home, exposure to vibration, even relatively low levels, can contribute to the development of CTS symptoms. This does not mean you need to avoid mowing the lawn or blow-drying your hair. Instead, be aware of your body, and if you start to experience symptoms suggestive of CTS, limit these activities.

Ͼ **Strengthen muscles.** The stronger your muscles are, the easier it is to keep your wrist supported in a neutral position. Good muscle strength ensures the ability to maintain proper form when performing activities, because when fatigue sets in, our technique breaks down. When our technique breaks down, we become more prone to injury—again a principle from athletics that applies to our musculoskeletal system in general. And importantly, the more we develop our muscles, the more we improve our metabolic efficiency.

Ͼ **Optimize ergonomic environment.** Carefully evaluate your work environment and make sure it matches your body type and work habits. Use adaptive devices where able to minimize repetition and reduce stress. Avoid awkward body positions and unnatural motions. You may benefit from a formal ergonomic evaluation at your place of work.

☾ **Stretch (both whole body and upper extremity).** Stretching increases blood flow to the body and relaxes your muscles. Getting in the habit of performing whole body stretches as well as extremity-focused stretches will decrease tension and stress on your musculoskeletal system. There is no perfect way to stretch, just focus on a muscle group and move until you feel it under gentle stretching tension. Hold the stretch gently for 20 to 30 seconds and then release. There is no need for aggressive motion or sudden movements. Go slow and let your body's tension release naturally.

MEDICAL CONDITIONS

Poor management of underlying medical conditions can worsen the symptoms of CTS and make them more difficult to treat. When a medical condition like diabetes is poorly managed, it increases the risk of developing associated conditions like CTS. As an example, treating an underactive thyroid and returning you to a normal thyroid state may reduce symptoms of CTS. Another medical condition strongly associated with the development of

CTS is obesity and weight loss will positively affect more than just your CTS.

Physical Activity & Metabolic Efficiency

Increasing your level of physical activity and optimizing your metabolic efficiency are often overlooked in the treatment of CTS. Optimizing your metabolic efficiency can reduce your risk of developing certain medical conditions or minimize the effect of those conditions. For example, one benefit of improving your body's metabolic efficiency is better glucose control, which is of importance for people with diabetes. Improved metabolic efficiency can also help to reduce inflammation both acute and chronic. When acute inflammation results in swelling of the tendon linings within the carpal tunnel, it creates a mass effect that puts pressure on the median nerve. Chronic inflammation is associated with many diseases (diabetes, obesity, heart disease, depression, cancer) and improving our metabolic efficiency is probably one of the most important things we can do to minimize the risk of developing these conditions. That means careful attention to sleep, diet, hydration, stress management and exercise. Finally, when we improve the metabolic efficiency of our bodies, we generally feel better, exercise is easier, and we begin to create a positively reinforcing cycle of experiences that builds our sense of self-efficacy.

YOUR HANDS

SPLINTING

We begin by splinting the wrist in the neutral position at night (see figure 41). This is a time-tested treatment that is supported by the best available evidence. If symptoms are persistent, the splint can also be worn during the day, but you may benefit from having the wrist in a more functional position for activities than the purely neutral night splint position. That would mean a second splint for day wear that has the wrist in about 15° of extension.

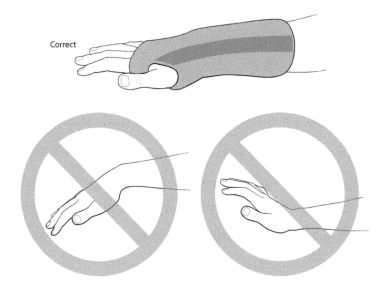

Figure 41
How to Wear a Splint for CTS
The proper wrist position when wearing a splint for CTS is with the wrist in the neutral position. Note that the wrist is neither flexed nor extended when the splint is positioned properly.

Nerve & Tendon Gliding Exercises

The other important thing that you can do for your hands is to perform nerve and tendon gliding exercises. These have been shown to increase the blood flow to the nerve and are associated with a decrease in symptoms when performed regularly.

Hand Therapy

Many patients with CTS benefit from visiting with a Hand Therapist. They can receive personalized instruction in how to perform nerve and tendon gliding exercise, including any necessary modifications based on their unique anatomy. Hand therapists who are also Certified Ergonomists can evaluate how you interact with your work environment and make recommendations for strategies to improve your function and adaptive equipment to decrease activity load. Well trained Hand Therapists will also evaluate your hand and wrist function in the context of your entire extremity to help minimize the risk of developing, and treat if present, associated conditions like elbow or wrist tendonitis.

YOUR DOCTOR

The final area of focus is Your Doctor. If you have worked through the You and Your Hands steps of the pathway and are still having symptoms of CTS, then the next step is to visit with your doctor.

An electrodiagnostic study will often be requested, and this has two important functions when considering your symptoms and urgency of treatment. First, it will help to identify other possible causes of the symptoms you are experiencing. For example, generalized peripheral neuropathy will look different on the electrodiagnostic study than CTS. The other important information it provides is an estimate of severity.

An electrodiagnostic study is not an absolute test for CTS. It requires interpretation in the context of your symptoms. If the test shows that the conduction delay is significantly elevated at the level of the carpal tunnel, then we know from experience that the chances of splinting, exercises, and injections helping are reduced. With this information, patients may elect to proceed with surgery and avoid prolonging their suffering and the associated negative impact on their productivity for another six to eight weeks.

After discussing all this information and your specific circumstances with your doctor, one of three paths will generally be followed: (1) do nothing, continue to monitor your symptoms;

(2) perform an injection and see if that resolves your symptoms; or (3) proceed to surgery to relieve the symptoms and fix the problem.

When you experience relief from the symptoms of numbness and tingling, you have reached a successful conclusion to treatment. Sometimes when my patients are unsure of their symptom relief or have symptoms and are not sure if they are ready for surgery, we will consider repeating the electrodiagnostic testing after a six-month period. This allows enough time to pass between tests for us to observe meaningful changes. If we repeat testing and the nerve conduction is worsening, then we know that the condition is not really improving, and patients can make an informed decision about their next step in treatment.

If you have followed the treatment pathway and your symptoms have resolved, congratulations! Now the next step will be to consider what you do going forward to either prevent the condition from happening in your other hand or from coming back in the same hand. That is the purpose of the HandGuyMD® CTS Prevention Pathway discussed in Appendix B.

Appendix B:

HANDGUYMD®
CTS PREVENTION PROGRAM

While there is no magic bullet or pill that will prevent CTS (or just about any disease for that matter), there are helpful actions that you can take with an eye toward prevention. The best evidence supports following the steps outlined in the HandGuyMD® CTS Prevention Program to minimize your risk of developing CTS.

As with the treatment of CTS, it is helpful to have a conceptual framework for thinking about the prevention of CTS. In Chapter 8, we discussed the CTS Prevention Staircase (see figure 42) and the conceptual framework for thinking about prevention builds off this foundation. You will notice that there is overlap between the treatment and prevention pathways, and that is for good reason. When the symptoms of CTS are reversible, the steps you take to reverse them become the same steps you need to keep taking to prevent the symptoms from coming back.

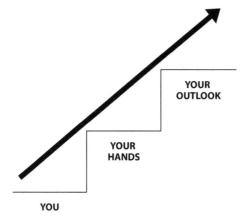

CARPAL TUNNEL PREVENTION "STAIRCASE"

Figure 42
The CTS Prevention Staircase
There are many factors that contribute to the possible prevention of CTS. One way to
organize the information is to think about the many parts as an ascending staircase that
progresses from You to Your Hands to Your Outlook. At each step along the way, you
can act to minimize the risk of CTS development and progression.

You

The first step in the prevention of CTS begins with You and
this means addressing your genetic makeup, general conditioning,
and management of medical conditions. You cannot alter your
genetic makeup and, fortunately, a genetic predisposition to
developing nerve compression syndromes like CTS is rare. The
effect of structural anomalies, like having small bones that make
for a narrow carpal tunnel or a low-lying tendon muscle belly that
enters the carpal tunnel, cannot be changed but their effects can be
minimized. The following areas, however, are under your control

and a proactive approach will reduce your risk developing CTS (see figure 43):

ℭ **General conditioning.** Improving your cardiovascular fitness reduces your risk of developing CTS and benefits your overall health no matter what your current level of activity. We know from the best evidence that increased physical activity appears to be associated with a lower risk of developing CTS. Furthermore, there is also strong evidence that increasing body weight is also associated with developing CTS. So, the more you can do to increase your physical activity and lose weight, the more likely you are to reduce your risk of developing CTS. The US Department of Health and Human Services Physical Activity Guidelines for Americans is a good starting point (see Table 15). Always consult your physician if you are starting a new exercise program.

TABLE 15
US HHS Physical Activity Guidelines for Americans

℃ 150 minutes of moderate intensity physical activity per week, OR

℃ 75 minutes of vigorous physical activity OR

℃ Equivalent combination (2 minutes of moderate = 1 minute of vigorous physical activity)

℃ Light activity is beneficial (in individuals performing no moderate to vigorous physical activity)

For more extensive health benefits:

℃ 300 minutes of moderate intensity physical activity OR

℃ 150 minutes of vigorous physical activity OR

℃ Equivalent combination

℃ Resistance training (muscle strengthening) at least twice per week

℃ **Management of Medical Conditions.** The next part of You to consider for prevention is your overall health and wellness. That means making sure that any medical conditions you may have are being appropriately managed. If your thyroid is not functioning properly, you may notice a reduction of your symptoms once it is correctly balanced. We can't really explain the direct link, but we do commonly see CTS symptoms in patients with certain medical conditions, and sometimes getting those conditions under control is associated with a reduction in symptoms. Also, in terms of prevention we want to minimize the risk of developing diabetes and obesity.

Chronic inflammation is associated with many diseases (diabetes, obesity, heart disease, depression, cancer) and improving our metabolic efficiency is probably one of the most important things we can do to minimize the risk of developing these conditions. That means careful attention to sleep, diet, hydration, stress management and exercise. When we improve the metabolic efficiency of our bodies, we generally feel better, exercise is easier, and we begin to create a positively reinforcing cycle of experiences that builds our sense of self-efficacy.

Finally, improving your metabolic efficiency supports you in your efforts to manage medical conditions, increase physical activity, and lose weight. After years of treating thousands of patients and studying the available evidence, I am convinced that this concept is going to be critical for keeping patients healthy and preventing much of the "disease" we are focused on treating in medicine.

Top 7 Health-related Carpal Tunnel Syndrome Prevention Tips

- INCREASE PHYSICAL ACTIVITY
- REDUCE BODYWEIGHT
- ENSURE PROPER MANAGEMENT OF MEDICAL CONDITIONS
- START NIGHT SPLINTING AT FIRST SIGN OF SYMPTOMS
- STRENGTHEN MUSCLES
- PERFORM NERVE AND TENDON GLIDING EXERCISES
- IMPROVE YOUR METABOLIC EFFICIENCY

Figure 43
Top 7 Health-Related CTS Prevention Tips
Our health affects our bodies in more ways than we realize. These tips will help to make sure your body is functioning at peak performance and minimize the risk of developing symptoms of CTS and other conditions.

YOUR HANDS

You need to consider the activities you perform and how you do them (see Figure 44).

Top 7 Activity-related Carpal Tunnel Syndrome Prevention Tips

- KEEP WRIST IN A NEUTRAL POSITION WHILE PERFORMING ACTIVITY
- USE PROPER GRIP TECHNIQUE
- MINIMIZE REPETITION WITH ACTIVITY
- REDUCE SPEED OF REPETITION WITH HAND USE
- REDUCE FORCE OF ACTIVITY WITH HAND USE
- LIMIT HAND EXPOSURE TO VIBRATION
- REST YOUR HANDS

Figure 44
Top 7 Activity-Related CTS Prevention Tips
When performing activities or working with your hands, these tips will help reduce the chances of developing symptoms, or minimize the severity of symptoms, associated with CTS.

With respect to activity modification, the following are important principles to keep in mind:

- **Keep your wrist in a neutral position.** When performing activities, try to avoid bending your wrist for prolonged periods.

- **Use proper grip technique.** Avoid gripping with just your fingertips and try to use your whole hand. Doing so allows you to engage larger muscles and minimize pinch force, which increases the pressure on the median nerve in the carpal tunnel.

- **Minimize repetition with activities.** Avoid forceful gripping and repetitive motion for long periods. If it can't be avoided, then be sure to take frequent breaks, switch hands, alternate tasks, minimize holding objects for long periods with your hand or wrist in the same position.

- **Rest your hands.** Take frequent breaks to avoid prolonged activity without changing hand or wrist position. When you are taking a break, be sure to do general stretching as well as nerve and tendon gliding exercises.

- **Reduce speed and force of activity.** When performing repetitive tasks, reducing both speed and force minimizes the risk of developing symptoms of CTS. You are allowing your body time to adjust to the activity and recover—think of yourself like an athlete who knows that continuous training will not allow for the needed rest that is critical for recovery between games. The same principle applies with our bodies—it is all about rest and recovery.

- Č **Limit the exposure of your hands to vibration**. At work or at home, exposure to vibration, even relatively low levels, can contribute to the development of CTS symptoms. This does not mean you need to avoid mowing the lawn or blow-drying your hair. Instead, be aware of your body, and if you start to experience symptoms suggestive of CTS, limit these activities.

- Č **Strengthen muscles.** The stronger your muscles are, the easier it is to keep your wrist supported in a neutral position. Good muscle strength ensures the ability to maintain proper form when performing activities, because when fatigue sets in, our technique breaks down. When our technique breaks down, we become more prone to injury—again a principle from athletics that applies to our musculoskeletal system in general. And importantly, the more we develop our muscles, the more we improve our metabolic efficiency.

Your ability to adhere to the principles outlined is affected by the ergonomic environment in which you operate. Making sure that the ergonomic environment is optimized is another important part of prevention. Putting your body in an optimal mechanical position to perform your tasks reduces the stress on your musculoskeletal system and minimizes the risk of overload. Finding alternate ways to perform repetitive tasks, using tools and automation and conscious design of the workflow will all reduce the burden on your musculoskeletal system.

YOUR OUTLOOK

Increasing your sense of self-efficacy and avoiding catastrophizing will reduce the chances of developing non-specific arm pain, which can be confused for CTS. When non-specific arm pain is present it is difficult to treat because the CTS treatments designed to address mechanical compression of the median nerve are not effective when the nerve is not under pressure.

Management of stress is vital and a technique that can improve both stress management as well as our overall metabolic efficiency is focused breathing. One method of focused breathing is to inhale for a count of "X", hold the breath for a count of "2X-4X" and then exhale for a count of "2X".

If you follow the steps outlined in the HandGuyMD® CTS Prevention Program you can be assured that you have done all that you can prevent the development of CTS. Will you always be successful? No, that is just a reality but the actions you take may very well be the difference between a condition that responds to nonoperative treatment and the need to have surgery.

REFERENCES

1. Luckhaupt SE, Dahlhamer JM, Ward BW, Sweeney MH, Sestito JP, Calver GM. 2013. "Prevalence and work-relatedness of carpal tunnel syndrome in the working population, United States, 2010 National Health Interview Survey." *Am J Ind Med* 56: 615-624.

2. Dale AM, Harris-Adamson C, Rempel D, et al. 2013. "Prevalence and incidence of carpal tunnel syndrome in US working populations: pooled analysis of six prospective studies." *Scand J Work Environ Health* 39 (5): 495-505.

3. Spinner RJ, Bachman JW, Amadio PC. 1989. "The many faces of carpal tunnel syndrome." *Mayo Clin Proc* 64: 829-36.

4. American Academy of Orthopedic Surgeons. 2008, revised 2011, 2016. *Clinical Practice Guideline on the Treatment of Carpal Tunnel Syndrome*. American Academy of Orthopedic Surgeons.

5. Watson-Jones R. 1929. "Carpal semilunar dislocations and other wrist dislocations with associated nerve lesions." *Proc Royal Soc Med* 22: 1071-86.

6. You D, Smith AH, Rempel D. 2014. "Meta-analysis: association between wrist posture and carpal tunnel syndrome among workers." *Saf Health Work* 5 (1): 27-31.

7. Paget J. 1854. *Lectures on Surgical Pathology*. Philadelphia: Lindsay & Blakiston.

8. Putnam J. 1880. A series of cases of paresthesia, mainly of the hands, of periodical recurrence, and possibly of vaso-motor origin. *Arch of Medicine (New York) 4: 147-62*.

9. Schultze F. 1893. "Uber Akroparasthesie." *Deutsche Zeitschrift fur Nervenheilkunde* (Deutsche Zeitschrift fur Nervenheilkunde) 3: 300-318.

10. Hunt JR. 1908. "Occupational neuritis of the thenar branch of the median nerve: a well-defined type of occupation atrophy of the hand." *The Journal of Nervous and Mental Disease* 35.

11. Marie P, Foix C. 1913. "Atrophie isolee de l'eminence thenar d'origine nevritique. Role du ligament annulaire du carpe dans la pathogenie de al lesion." *Rev Neurol* 26: 647-649.

12. Lewis D, Miller EM. 1922. "Peripheral nerve injuries associated with fractures." *Ann Surg* 76: 528-538.

13. Abbott LC, Saunders JB del M. 1933. "Injuries of the median nerve in fractures of the lower end of the radius." *Surg Gynecol Obstet* 57: 507-516.

14. Amadio PC. 1995. "The first carpal tunnel release?" *J Hand Surg Am 20 (1): 40-41.*

15. Learmonth JR. 1933. "The principle of decompression in the treatment of certain diseases of peripheral nerves." *Surg Clin N Am* 13: 905-13.

16. Moersch FP. 1938. "Median thenar neuritis." *Proceedings of the Staff Meetings of the Mayo Clinic* 13: 220-22.

17. Brain WR, Wright AD, Wilkinson M. 1947. "Spontaneous compression of both median nerves in the carpal tunnel: six cases treated surgically." *Lancet* 1: 277-82.

18. Phalen GS. Gardner WJ, LaLonde AA. 1950. "Neuropathy of the median nerve due to compression beneath the transverse carpal ligament." *J Bone Joint Surg* 32A: 109-112.

19. Phalen GS. 1951. "Spontaneous compression of the median nerve at the wrist." *JAMA* 145: 1128-33.

20. Palmer DH, Hanrahan LP. 1995. *Social and economic costs of carpal tunnel surgery.* Instructional Course Lectures. Edited by Jackson DW. St. Louis: Mosby.

21. Atroshi I, England M, Turkiewicz A, Tagil M, Petersson IF. 2011. "Incidence of physician-diagnosed carpal tunnel syndrome in the general population." *Arch Intern Med* 171 (10): 943-944.

22. Hagberg M, Morgentsern H, Kelsh M. 1992. "Impact of occupations and job tasks on the prevalence of carpal tunnel syndrome." *Scand J Work Environ Health* 18 (6): 337-45.

23. Bagatur AE, Zorer G. 2001. "The carpal tunnel syndrome is a bilateral disorder." *J Bone Joint Surg Br* 83 (5): 655-658.

24. Fajardo M, Kim SH, Szabo RM. 2012. "Incidence of carpal tunnel release: trends and implications within the United States ambulatory care setting." *J Hand Surg Am* 37 (8): 1599-1605.

25. Fowler JR. 2014. "Endoscopic carpal tunnel release." *UPMC Dept Ortho Surg, Restore 1-2, 6.*

26. Hales TR, Bernard BP. 1996. "Epidemiology of work-related musculoskeletal disorders." *Ortho Clin N Amer* 27: 679-709.

27. Anderson JS, Thomsen JF, Overgaaard E, Lassen CF, Brandt LPA, Vilstrup I, Kryger AI, Mikkelsen S. 2003. "Computer use and carpal tunnel syndrome: a 1-year follow-up study." *JAMA 289: 2963-2969.*

28. Stevens C, Finsen L, Sogaard K, Christensen H. 2001. "The frequency of carpal tunnel syndrome in computer users at a medical facility." *Neurology* 56: 1568-1570.

29. Industrial Insurance Medical Advisory Committee [Upper Extremity Entrapment Neuropathies]. 2009. *Medical Treatment Guidelines. Work-Related Carpal Tunnel Syndrome. Diagnosis and Treatment Guideline.* Olympia, WA: Washington State Department of Labor and Industries.

30. Prakash KM, Fook-Chong S, Leoh TH, Dan YF, Nurjannah S, Tan YE, Lo, YL. 2006. "Sensitivities of sensory nerve conduction study parameters in carpal tunnel syndrome." *J Clin Neurophysiol* 23 (6): 565-567.

31. Grundberg AB. 1983. "Carpal tunnel decompression in spite of normal electromyography." *J Hand Surg Am* 8: 348-9.

32. Watson J, Zhao M, Ring D. 2010. "Predictors of normal electrodiagnostic testing in the evaluation of suspected carpal tunnel syndrome." *J Hand Microsurg 2 (2): 47-50.*

33. Lo JK, Finestone HM, Gilbert K, Woodbury MG. 2002. "Community-based referrals for electrodiagnostic studies in patients with possible carpal tunnel syndrome: what is the diagnosis?" *Arch Phys Med Rehabil* 83: 598-603.

34. Schrijver HM, Gerritsen AA, Strijers RL, et al. 2005. "Correlating nerve conduction studies and clinical outcome measures on carpal tunnel syndrome: lessons from a randomized controlled trial." *J Clin Neurophysiol* 22: 216-21.

35. Leighton C, Turner JA, Comstock BA, Levenson LM, Hollingworth W, Heagerty PJ, Kliot M, Jarvik JG. 2007. "The relationship between electrodiagnostic findings and patient symptoms and function in carpal tunnel syndrome." *Arch Phys Med Rehabil* 88: 19-24.

36. Dhong ES, Han SK, Lee BI, Kim WK. 2000. "Correlation of electrodiagnostic findings with subjective symptoms in carpal tunnel syndrome." *Ann Plast Surg* 45 (2): 127-31.

37. Rozmaryn LM, Dovelle S, Rothman ER, Gorman K, Olvey KM, Barko JJ. 1998. "Nerve and tendon gliding exercises and the conservative management of carpal tunnel syndrome." *Journal Hand Therapy* July-Sept: 171-79.

38. Edgell SE, McCabe SJ, Breidenbach WC, LaJoie AS, Abell TD. 2003. "Predicting the outcome of carpal tunnel release." *J Hand Surg Am* 28: 255-61.

39. Zhang S, Vora M, Harris AHS, Baker L, Curtin C, Kamal RN. 2016. "Cost-minimization analysis of open and endoscopic carpal tunnel release." *J Bone Joint Surg Am* 98: 1970-1977.

40. Vasen AP, Kuntz KM, Simmons BP, Katz JN. 1999. "Open versus endoscopic carpal tunnel release: a decision analysis." *J Hand Surg Am* 24 (5): 1109-17.

41. Park KW, Boyer MI, Gelberman RH, Calfee RP, Stepan JG, Osei DA. 2016. "Simultaneous bilateral versus staged bilateral carpal tunnel release: A Cost-effectiveness Analysis." *J Am Acad Orthop Surg* 24: 796-804.

42. Bogunovic L, Gelberman RH, Goldfarb CA, Boyer MI, Calfee BP. 2013. "The impact of antiplatelet medication on hand and wrist surgery." *J Hand Surg Am 38 (6): 1063-70.*

43. Bobunovic L, Gelberman RH, Goldfarb CA, Boyer MI, Calfee BP. 2015. "The impact of uninterrupted warfarin on hand and wrist surgery." *J Hand Surg Am 40 (11): 2133-40.*

44. Miller A, Kim N, Zmistowski B, Ilyas AM, Matzon JL. 2017. "Postoperative pain management following carpal tunnel release: A prospective cohort evaluation." *Hand* 12 (6): 541-45.

45. Phillips EM. 2018. "The Exercise Prescription." June 23.

46. United States Department of Health and Human Services. 2008. "health.gov." *Physical Activity Guidelines for Americans.* October 1. https://health.gov/paguidelines/pdf/paguide.pdf.

47. Phillips EM. 2018. "Draft Update US HHS Physical Activity Guidelines." June 23.

48. Chabok HA, Ring D. 2014. "Arm ache." *HAND* 9(2): 151-155.

49. Rabasa C, Dickson SL. 2016. "Impact of stress on metabolism and energy balance." *Current Opinion in Behavioral Sciences* 9: 71-77.

50. Carayon P, Haims MC, Smith MJ. 1999. "Work organizations, job stress and work-related musculoskeletal disorders." *Human Factors* 41: 644-663.

GLOSSARY OF TERMS

Anesthesia doctor—The doctor who is responsible for the administration and monitoring of your anesthesia during and after surgery.

Atrophy—Muscle wasting that results from lack of use. This can occur either when the nerve that supplies the muscle is damaged and thus cannot send messages to the muscle (as in CTS), or when the muscle is immobilized to prevent its use (for example, to protect a healing injury).

Bier block—A form of intravenous regional anesthesia that is frequently used for upper extremity surgery. It renders the affected limb numb, allowing for surgery to proceed and does not have the risks associated with general anesthesia.

Brachial plexus—A network of nerves formed from parts of the lower cervical (neck) nerves and the first thoracic (chest) nerve. The collection of nerves is rearranged within the brachial plexus, and they emerge to enter the arm as the major named nerves in the extremity (radial, median, ulnar, musculocutaneous).

Catastrophizing—To imagine the worst possible outcome of an action or event.

Circulating nurse—The member of the surgery team who is responsible for the part of the operating room that is not sterile. They are the quarterback of the OR team, making sure everything is in its place and communicating with both the pre- and post-anesthesia care teams about the case.

Cognitive behavioral therapy—A type of psychotherapy in which negative patterns of thought about the self and the world are challenged to alter unwanted behavior patterns or treat a wide range of problems. It results in increased happiness by modifying dysfunctional emotions, behaviors, and thoughts.

Dose response effect—The idea that the greater your exposure to the risk factor, the greater the risk of developing CTS. Little exposure, little risk and high exposure, high risk. This is a fundamental criterion for establishing causality in medicine.

Ergonomic environments—Refers to the space in which you work and how it is set up in relation to your body. It includes the equipment you use, how it is used (for example, repetitive or prolonged use), how your body is positioned during that use.

Focused breathing—A technique for mindful breathing where individuals focus their attention on their breath, from inhale to a brief hold to exhale. It makes breathing the focus of concentration.

Generalizability—The concept that the results of a study using a sample of the population can be thought of as representing the results you would observe if you studied the whole population from which the sample was drawn. This is an important concept in science because if you have a flawed study based on a sample, you cannot then apply those results to everybody.

History—The process by which a doctor gathers information from you about your condition and what has been happening up until the time of your visit.

Hypothesis—An idea, or proposed explanation, developed based on limited information that explains an observation and serves as the starting point for further investigation. In medicine, the description of your symptoms (observation) is the limited information we use to develop a hypothesis, which we further test with additional questions, a physical examination and diagnostic testing.

Idiopathic—How we describe a disease condition that arises spontaneously or for which the cause is unknown.

Incidence—The frequency with which a disease occurs in a population.

Median—I know it is confusing but this does not refer to the median nerve! Median is a statistical term that defines the specific value within a data set at which 50% of the values within the data set are above the "median" and 50% are below. The use of a median avoids the possible skewing that can occur when an average is used and there are values at either extreme of the range for the data set.

Median nerve—One of three major nerves that supply the hand. It provides sensation for the thumb, index, middle, and one-half of the ring finger.

NPO—Latin for "nils per os," which means "nothing by mouth." This is meant literally with respect to surgery. We do not want you to have any food or drink before surgery.

Odds-ratio—A measure of the association between an exposure (think of risk factor) and an outcome. The odds-ratio tells you the odds (or chances) that an outcome will occur given a specific exposure, compared to the odds (or chances) that the same outcome would occur without the specific exposure. For example, an odds-ratio of 3 for keyboarding means that you are three times more likely to develop CTS if you keyboard than if you did not keyboard.

Paresthesias—Abnormal sensations, often described as a prickling or tingling feeling (pins and needles), because of pressure on, or damage to, a peripheral nerve.

Pathophysiology—The physiological processes that are disordered, or not functioning properly, with a disease or injury.

Peripheral nerve entrapment neuropathy—Just a fancy way to say that a nerve is pinched somewhere after it leaves the spinal cord. Usually, this pinching occurs somewhere along the nerves, as it travels within the arm or leg.

Phalen's sign—A physical exam test for carpal tunnel syndrome in which the patient flexes both wrists. Phalen's sign is said to be "positive" if the patient develops numbness or tingling in the median nerve distribution within sixty seconds.

Presurgery nurse—The nurse who will be taking care of you before you enter the operating room. They are the first member of the surgery team you will meet on the day of surgery.

Prevalence—The percentage of the population that is affected by a disease condition at a certain point in time.

Scrub nurse—The member of the surgery team who is responsible for the instruments used during surgery. Their "back table" has all the sterile instruments, and the scrub nurse gives the instruments to the surgeon as they are needed during the surgery. They play an important role on the surgery team and by anticipating the next step in a surgery can make the case flow smoothly.

Self-efficacy—Refers to people's belief about their ability to produce specific levels of performance. It describes a confidence in our ability to exert control over our own motivation, behavior, and social environment.

Sensitivity—Refers to the ability of a test to correctly identify someone who has the condition the test is supposed to identify (a true positive).

Signs—Objective evidence of a disease condition identified by direct physical examination of the patient.

Specificity—Refers to the ability of a test to correctly identify those who do not have the condition the test is supposed to identify (a true negative).

Synergistic relationship—The idea that while the risk of developing CTS in the presence of any one individual risk factor may be small, when you start to add two or more risk factors, the relative risk of developing CTS is greater than the sum of the individual risks. In other words, 1+1 > 2.

Symptoms—Subjective evidence suggesting the presence of a disease condition that is reported by the patient.

Tardy median nerve palsy—The term used when the onset of median nerve dysfunction is delayed or occurs sometime later after an injury.

Tendonopathies—A general term that refers to disorders affecting tendons, including acute injury (from overuse) and chronic injury that is not healed. These disorders can occur anywhere along the tendon but are most common where the tendon originates and where the tendon attaches to bone.

Tinel's sign—A way to identify nerves that are irritated. The examiner "taps" over the nerve and, if it is positive, the patient will feel a tingling sensation along the distribution of the nerve.

Validity—Tells us how well a test measures what it is intended to measure.

INDEX

Abbott, 22
abductor pollicis brevis muscle 6, 43, 46, 48, 61-2, 68-9, 90, 124
acroparesthesia 20
APB see abductor pollicis brevis muscle
arm ache 71-3, 159-61, 165, 167-8

bier block anesthesia 102, 105, 108-9, 110-12, 114, 120, 211
Body Mass Index (BMI) 7, 12, 60
brachial plexus 17, 20, 58, 209

carpal tunnel
    anatomy 4
carpal tunnel syndrome
    diagnosis see diagnosis, carpal tunnel syndrome
    dynamic 74
    idiopathic 6, 43, 58, 212
    incidence 10, 28, 31, 152, 212
    natural history 42-3, 47-8, 90
    pregnancy 8, 42, 56
    prevalence 3, 6, 11-12, 28, 41, 216
    recurrent 128, 131-2
    risk factors 7-9, 12, 30-34, 41, 61,
    aging 29
    dose response effect 31, 212
    occupation 6, 12, 28-31, 35, 41, 131, 152
    odds-ratio 30, 213
    physical activity 10, 34, 80, 148-50, 181, 185, 192-5

splinting 19, 25, 80, 82, 87-8, 91, 98, 152, 161, 173, 181, 186, 188, 195
surgery see surgery, carpal tunnel syndrome
treatment program 179

catastrophizing 169, 174, 198, 210
chronic stress 168
CHT see hand therapy, certified hand therapist
Clinical Practice Guideline 4, 6, 37, 39, 41, 61, 79, 82-85, 133, 176
cognitive behavioral therapy 161, 169, 210
coping skill 160-61
CTS see carpal tunnel syndrome

diagnosis, carpal tunnel syndrome
    conditions that may look like CTS 58
    electrodiagnostically negative CTS 69-70
    electrodiagnostic testing 15, 66, 75, 80, 181, 189
    flick test 55-6, 61
    history 54, 59-61, 63-4, 72, 211
    Phalen's sign (test) 25-6, 63, 213
    physical exam tests 62-3
    physical signs 61, 215
    atrophy of APB 5-6, 43-4, 48, 61-2
    physician's intuition 71-2, 74
    questionnaires 58-9, 75

prevention 144-47, 174-5, 189-99
prevention conceptual staircase 174, 190
prevention program 144, 175, 190
rest 33, 154-5, 157, 174, 181-3, 195-7,
US Health and Human Services Physical Activity Guidelines for Americans 149, 192
top 7 activity-related prevention tips 195
top 7 health-related prevention tips 195
vibration 8, 34, 64, 154, 174, 183, 195, 197
Putnam, James 19-20
Putnam's paresthesia 20

Schultze, Fredrich 20
self-efficacy 159-62, 164-9, 174, 185, 194-5, 198, 214
splinting 19, 25, 80, 82, 87-8, 91. 98, 152, 173, 181, 186, 195
steroid
injection 70, 72, 80, 87-8, 91, 98, 181
oral 85-6
surgery, carpal tunnel syndrome 44, 46, 68, 70, 72, 80, 87-98, 99, 105-7, 112-14, 119, 123, 125, 131, 135-8, 176, 181
anesthesia doctor 101, 105-11, 209
antibiotics 112-14
conversion-to-open 93-4
dividing transverse carpal ligament 23-4, 90, 116-18, 124
endoscopic 91-4, 97-8, 114, 116-18
medicines before 100, 103-5
NPO 101-3, 212
nurse
circulating 101, 106-8, 111, 139, 210
presurgery 105-6, 214
scrub 107-8, 111, 139, 214

open 23, 27, 91-94, 98, 132
post anesthesia care unit (PACU) 120
postoperative dressing 119, 123, 126
simultaneous (bilateral) 95-7
staged 95-7
time out 112-13

thenar muscle atrophy 6, 20, 62
thoracic outlet syndrome 17, 58, 72
transverse carpal ligament (anatomy) 4

WALANT (wide awake local anesthesia no tourniquet) 111
Watson-Jones 22
wellness 80, 181, 193
inflammation 150-1, 168, 174, 185, 194
metabolic efficiency 80, 170, 181, 183, 185, 194-5, 197-8

ABOUT THE AUTHOR

W ren V. McCallister, MD, MBA has been practicing Hand Surgery in Edmonds, Washington since 2006. Board-certified in both Orthopedics and Hand Surgery, he has been recognized for excellence in patient care with numerous "Top Doctor" awards including Seattle Met Magazine and Castle Connolly. His award-winning work in clinical and basic science research has been published in the *Journal of Hand Surgery, Hand Clinics of North America, Journal of the American Academy of Orthopedic Surgeons, Orthopedic Clinics of North America, Journal of Bone and Joint Surgery, Journal of Reconstructive Microsurgery, Neurosurgery Clinics of North America, and Clinical Orthopaedics and Related Research.* Dr. McCallister is a Fellow of the American Academy of Orthopedic Surgery and is an Active Member of the American Society for Surgery of the Hand and American Association for Hand Surgery.

Dr. McCallister's focus now is on providing access to expert information and education that increases understanding of complex medical and surgical conditions affecting the hand and upper extremity. The **HandGuyMD® Patient Guide** series and **HandGuyMD.com** provide the same clear, concise, and understandable information his patients have benefited from and appreciated. **HandGuyMD®** is *"Expert Help for Hand Problems"*.

CPSIA information can be obtained
at www.ICGtesting.com
Printed in the USA
BVHW041048220222
629765BV00017B/674

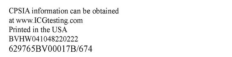

9 781662 842627